Natural Compounds as New Cancer Treatments

Natural Compounds as New Cancer Treatments

Special Issue Editor

Enrique Barrajón-Catalán

MDPI • Basel • Beijing • Wuhan • Barcelona • Belgrade

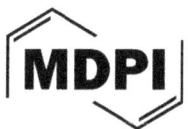

Special Issue Editor
Enrique Barrajón-Catalán
Universitas Miguel Hernández
Spain

Editorial Office
MDPI
St. Alban-Anlage 66
4052 Basel, Switzerland

This is a reprint of articles from the Special Issue published online in the open access journal *Medicines* (ISSN 2305-6320) from 2018 to 2019 (available at: https://www.mdpi.com/journal/medicines/special_issues/natural_compounds)

For citation purposes, cite each article independently as indicated on the article page online and as indicated below:

LastName, A.A.; LastName, B.B.; LastName, C.C. Article Title. *Journal Name* **Year**, *Article Number*, Page Range.

ISBN 978-3-03921-365-8 (Pbk)
ISBN 978-3-03921-366-5 (PDF)

Cover image courtesy of María Herranz-López.

© 2019 by the authors. Articles in this book are Open Access and distributed under the Creative Commons Attribution (CC BY) license, which allows users to download, copy and build upon published articles, as long as the author and publisher are properly credited, which ensures maximum dissemination and a wider impact of our publications.
The book as a whole is distributed by MDPI under the terms and conditions of the Creative Commons license CC BY-NC-ND.

Contents

About the Special Issue Editor vii

Enrique Barrajón-Catalán
Natural Compounds as New Cancer Treatments
Reprinted from: *Medicines* **2019**, *6*, 78, doi:10.3390/medicines6030078 . . . . **1**

Tung-chin Chiang, Brian Koss, L. Joseph Su, Charity L. Washam, Stephanie D. Byrum, Aaron Storey and Alan J. Tackett
Effect of Sulforaphane and 5-Aza-2′-Deoxycytidine on Melanoma Cell Growth
Reprinted from: *Medicines* **2019**, *6*, 71, doi:10.3390/medicines6030071 . . . . **4**

Kyohei Araki, Yasuyoshi Miyata, Kojiro Ohba, Yuichiro Nakamura, Tomohiro Matsuo, Yasushi Mochizuki and Hideki Sakai
Oral Intake of Royal Jelly Has Protective Effects Against Tyrosine Kinase Inhibitor-Induced Toxicity in Patients with Renal Cell Carcinoma: A Randomized, Double-Blinded, Placebo-Controlled Trial
Reprinted from: *Medicines* **2019**, *6*, 2, doi:10.3390/medicines6010002 . . . . **22**

Anh V. Le, Tien T. Huynh, Sophie E. Parks, Minh H. Nguyen and Paul D. Roach
Bioactive Composition, Antioxidant Activity, and Anticancer Potential of Freeze-Dried Extracts from Defatted Gac (*Momordica cochinchinensis* Spreng) Seeds
Reprinted from: *Medicines* **2018**, *5*, 104, doi:10.3390/medicines5030104 . . . . **33**

Mohd Farhan, Mohammad Fahad Ullah, Mohd Faisal, Ammad Ahmad Farooqi, Uteuliyev Yerzhan Sabitaliyevich, Bernhard Biersack and Aamir Ahmad
Differential Methylation and Acetylation as the Epigenetic Basis of Resveratrol's Anticancer Activity
Reprinted from: *Medicines* **2019**, *6*, 24, doi:10.3390/medicines6010024 . . . . **51**

María Herranz-López, María Losada-Echeberría and Enrique Barrajón-Catalán
The Multitarget Activity of Natural Extracts on Cancer: Synergy and Xenohormesis
Reprinted from: *Medicines* **2019**, *6*, 6, doi:10.3390/medicines6010006 . . . . **63**

Robert Hendler and Yue Zhang
Probiotics in the Treatment of Colorectal Cancer
Reprinted from: *Medicines* **2018**, *5*, 101, doi:10.3390/medicines5030101 . . . . **73**

Yasuyoshi Miyata, Tomohiro Matsuo, Kyohei Araki, Yuichiro Nakamura, Yuji Sagara, Kojiro Ohba and Hideki Sakai
Anticancer Effects of Green Tea and the Underlying Molecular Mechanisms in Bladder Cancer
Reprinted from: *Medicines* **2018**, *5*, 87, doi:10.3390/medicines5030087 . . . . **87**

Jean-Jacques Michaille, Victoria Piurowski, Brooke Rigot, Hesham Kelani, Emily C. Fortman and Esmerina Tili
MiR-663, a MicroRNA Linked with Inflammation and Cancer That Is under the Influence of Resveratrol
Reprinted from: *Medicines* **2018**, *5*, 74, doi:10.3390/medicines5030074 . . . . **105**

About the Special Issue Editor

Enrique Barrajón-Catalán was born in Madrid, Spain (1977) and obtained his degree in Biochemistry (1999) and Pharmacy (2011) from Miguel Hernández University (Elche, Spain). Here, he also obtained his PhD in Molecular and Cellular Biology in 2005. During his postdoctoral period (2006–2011), he worked at several companies researching natural compounds, and joined the staff of the Miguel Hernández University in 2011, where he became Professor in the Pharmacy and Pharmaceutical Technology Area, and Researcher at Instituto de Investigación Desarrollo e Innovación en Biotecnología Sanitaria de Elche (IDiBE). His research interests include the pharmacological activities of natural compounds, with special focus on cosmetics, obesity and metabolic syndrome, new antimicrobial development, and anticancer research.

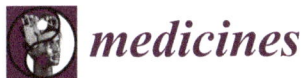

Editorial

Natural Compounds as New Cancer Treatments

Enrique Barrajón-Catalán

Instituto de Biología Molecular y Celular (IBMC) and Instituto de Investigación, Desarrollo e Innovación en Biotecnología Sanitaria de Elche (IDiBE), Universitas Miguel Hernández (UMH), 03202 Elche, Spain; e.barrajon@umh.es

Received: 15 July 2019; Accepted: 22 July 2019; Published: 23 July 2019

Cancer is still a global challenge worldwide with a high impact not only on human health, causing morbidity and mortality, but also on economics. Although significant advances have been obtained in early diagnosis and in the development of new drugs, there is still a need of new molecules that contribute to span and improve the actual therapeutic strategies.

Natural compounds from animal, microbial, vegetal, or fungi origin represent countless sources of new compounds that can be used as anticancer drugs if their activity, bioavailability, and toxicity are adequate. There are some general [1] and specific [2] reviews covering this topic, however, the use of natural compounds is not always supported by scientific evidence. This special issue tries to solve this problem, incorporating original manuscripts with new evidence on the use of natural compounds in cancer research and covering the actual state of the art with several reviews.

In this special issue original research manuscripts including both pure compounds and whole natural extracts have been included. Chiang et al. [3] have used sulforaphane, natural molecules previously characterized as promising for fighting cancer [4], to challenge melanoma in combination with the epigenetic drug 5-aza-2′-deoxycytidine (DAC). In this manuscript, the authors have observed that the combination between DAC and sulforaphane reduces melanoma cell growth by changing gene expression profiles but without altering epigenetics. This manuscript is relevant as it demonstrates that the ingestion of some natural compounds can improve the outcome of some cancer treatments. In this sense, this relationship between diet and drugs is not new [5]. There is a long list of interactions between foods and drugs, but these results must be taken in mind carefully as the interactions will not always be beneficious and every case must be studied individually and in the context of a complete and balanced diet. In addition, studies about natural compounds' bioavailability must also be done to ensure that the dose of the natural compounds that can influence drug treatments is achieved.

This special issue also contains data on the use of whole extracts and complex mixtures. Araki et al. [6] present their results about the use of royal jelly from honey bees on a randomized, double-blind, placebo-controlled trial. Royal jelly is a well-known functional food with relevant health-promoting properties [7]. In their manuscript, Araki et al. focus on patients with renal cell carcinoma under tyrosine kinase inhibitors treatment and observed that those who were supplemented with royal jelly presented lower side effect levels in terms of fatigue and anorexia. This clinical trial does not pretend to introduce royal jelly as an anticancer treatment, but suggests its use as a complementary treatment that could be useful to treat side effects of tyrosine kinase inhibitors treatment. However, further studies increasing the obtained evidence would be interesting before recommending its use in cancer patients, especially those focused on the putative interference between the compounds and the pharmacological treatments.

The last original manuscript of this special issue also studies a complex mixture of natural compounds. Le et al. studied the anticancer potential of a whole natural extract obtained from *Momordica cochinensis* seeds [8]. They performed different extraction procedures and studied the correlation between main compound families and antioxidant, and anticancer activities using different statistical approaches. This is a preliminary study that can be a first step for the future use of these extracts for melanoma treatment research, but before that, a whole extract characterization must be done in order to ensure which compounds are present qualitatively and quantitatively. In addition, expanding the research to other cancer types would be also recommendable.

Reviews are also included in this special issue covering different topics with significant relevance regarding cancer research. Two of these reviews are focused on the pure compound resveratrol. Resveratrol is a stilbene with a long list of biological activities [9], including cardiovascular disease prevention [10], UV protection [11], antiobesity [12], and anticancer properties [13,14]. The first review about resveratrol resumes the actual evidence on the epigenetic changes induced by resveratrol in the context of cancer [15]. It underlines the evidence about the epigenetic action of resveratrol on different types of cancer, including breast, lung, cervical, colon, leukemia, lymphoma, and prostate cancers, providing interesting comments about the existing evidence on each case. The second review about resveratrol is more specific, as it focuses on the role of resveratrol in the expression of the miR-663 microRNA and the relationships between this expression, inflammation, and cancer [16].

Green tea polyphenols have been also reviewed in this special issue. Miyata et al. [17] present in their review an extensive study of the anticancer effects of these polyphenols against bladder cancer. They cover not only in vitro studies using bladder cancer cell lines and in vivo studies using animal models but also new treatment strategies for patients with bladder cancer, based on green tea consumption.

Probiotics are also included in this special issue. Hendler et al. [18] update the previously published evidence on the relationship between probiotics and colon cancer [19,20]. They have written their review with a special interest on animal and human studies. They conclude that the use of probiotics can be recommended to reduce the colon cancer risk by influencing the microbiome composition. However, a more ambitious study, like a metanalysis must be done to reinforce this conclusion.

A global perspective on the use of natural compounds in cancer treatment is taken by Herranz et al. in their review [21]. In this manuscript, the authors provide an interesting point of view about the relevance of multitargeting and synergy when studying natural compounds. The molecular promiscuity of natural compounds has also been discussed by the same authors [22], but in this manuscript they focus on cancer, providing advice on experiment design and presenting the advantages and drawbacks when using complex mixtures of natural compounds as extracts. This last point is especially relevant, as there are still some points that must be improved in natural compounds research if we aspire to be considered as seriously as other disciplines are. As mentioned in this review, correct identification of the compounds, extract reproducibility, and bioavailability studies are the main but not the only weal points of natural product research. Better designs for in vivo trials, the use of non-tumor cell lines as controls of in vitro experiments, and synergy studies with other natural and non-natural compounds, especially clinically used drugs, will be welcome.

Finally, this special issue has met its original objective, contributing to increase the scientific evidence on the use of natural compounds in cancer research and treatment. However, there is a long way ahead, and new studies and evidence must be obtained in the future. Nature is a limitless source of new drugs, but these new drugs must always be supported by strong scientific evidence.

Funding: This research was funded by project RTI2018-096724-B-C21 from the Spanish Ministerio de Ciencia, Innovación y Universidades and project, PROMETEO/2016/006 from Generalitat Valenciana (Spain).

Conflicts of Interest: The authors declare no conflict of interest.

References

1. Fresco, P.; Borges, F.; Diniz, C.; Marques, M.P. New insights on the anticancer properties of dietary polyphenols. *Med. Res. Rev.* **2006**, *26*, 747–766. [CrossRef] [PubMed]
2. Losada-Echeberria, M.; Herranz-Lopez, M.; Micol, V.; Barrajon-Catalan, E. Polyphenols as promising drugs against main breast cancer signatures. *Antioxidants* **2017**, *6*, 88. [CrossRef] [PubMed]
3. Chiang, T.-C.; Koss, B.; Su, L.J.; Washam, C.L.; Byrum, S.D.; Storey, A.; Tackett, A.J. Effect of sulforaphane and 5-aza-2′-deoxycytidine on melanoma cell growth. *Medicines* **2019**, *6*, 71. [CrossRef] [PubMed]

4. Lenzi, M.; Fimognari, C.; Hrelia, P. Sulforaphane as a promising molecule for fighting cancer. *Cancer Treat. Res.* **2014**, *159*, 207–223. [PubMed]
5. Guo, W.; Kong, E.; Meydani, M. Dietary polyphenols, inflammation, and cancer. *Nutr. Cancer* **2009**, *61*, 807–810. [CrossRef] [PubMed]
6. Araki, K.; Miyata, Y.; Ohba, K.; Nakamura, Y.; Matsuo, T.; Mochizuki, Y.; Sakai, H. Oral intake of royal jelly has protective effects against tyrosine kinase inhibitor-induced toxicity in patients with renal cell carcinoma: A randomized, double-blinded, placebo-controlled trial. *Medicines* **2018**, *6*, 2. [CrossRef]
7. Ramadan, M.F.; Al-Ghamdi, A. Bioactive compounds and health-promoting properties of royal jelly: A review. *J. Funct. Foods* **2012**, *4*, 39–52. [CrossRef]
8. Le, A.V.; Huynh, T.T.; Parks, S.E.; Nguyen, M.H.; Roach, P.D. Bioactive composition, antioxidant activity, and anticancer potential of freeze-dried extracts from defatted gac (momordica cochinchinensis spreng) seeds. *Medicines* **2018**, *5*, 104. [CrossRef]
9. Tyagi, S.; Singh, G.; Sharma, A.; Aggarwal, G. Clinical and medicinal applications of resveratrol: A review. *Int. J. Pharm. Sci. Rev. Res.* **2010**, *3*, 49–52.
10. Das, S.; Das, D.K. Resveratrol: A therapeutic promise for cardiovascular diseases. *Recent Pat. Cardiovasc. Drug Discov.* **2007**, *2*, 133–138.
11. Park, K.; Lee, J.H. Protective effects of resveratrol on uvb-irradiated hacat cells through attenuation of the caspase pathway. *Oncol. Rep.* **2008**, *19*, 413–417. [CrossRef] [PubMed]
12. Eseberri, I.; Lasa, A.; Churruca, I.; Portillo, M.P. Resveratrol metabolites modify adipokine expression and secretion in 3t3-l1 pre-adipocytes and mature adipocytes. *PLoS ONE* **2013**, *8*, e63918. [CrossRef] [PubMed]
13. Bishayee, A. Cancer prevention and treatment with resveratrol: From rodent studies to clinical trials. *Cancer Prev. Res.* **2009**, *2*, 409–418. [CrossRef] [PubMed]
14. Catania, A.; Barrajon-Catalan, E.; Nicolosi, S.; Cicirata, F.; Micol, V. Immunoliposome encapsulation increases cytotoxic activity and selectivity of curcumin and resveratrol against her2 overexpressing human breast cancer cells. *Breast Cancer Res. Treat.* **2013**, *141*, 55–65. [CrossRef] [PubMed]
15. Farhan, M.; Ullah, M.F.; Faisal, M.; Farooqi, A.A.; Sabitaliyevich, U.Y.; Biersack, B.; Ahmad, A. Differential methylation and acetylation as the epigenetic basis of resveratrol's anticancer activity. *Medicines* **2019**, *6*, 24. [CrossRef]
16. Michaille, J.-J.; Piurowski, V.; Rigot, B.; Kelani, H.; Fortman, E.C.; Tili, E. Mir-663, a microrna linked with inflammation and cancer that is under the influence of resveratrol. *Medicines* **2018**, *5*, 74. [CrossRef]
17. Miyata, Y.; Matsuo, T.; Araki, K.; Nakamura, Y.; Sagara, Y.; Ohba, K.; Sakai, H. Anticancer effects of green tea and the underlying molecular mechanisms in bladder cancer. *Medicines* **2018**, *5*, 87. [CrossRef]
18. Hendler, R.; Zhang, Y. Probiotics in the treatment of colorectal cancer. *Medicines* **2018**, *5*, 101. [CrossRef]
19. Rafter, J. Probiotics and colon cancer. *Bailliere's Best Pract. Res. Clin. Gastroenterol.* **2003**, *17*, 849–859. [CrossRef]
20. Wollowski, I.; Rechkemmer, G.; Pool-Zobel, B.L. Protective role of probiotics and prebiotics in colon cancer. *Am. J. Clin. Nutr.* **2001**, *73*, 451S–455S. [CrossRef]
21. Herranz-López, M.; Losada-Echeberría, M.; Barrajón-Catalán, E. The multitarget activity of natural extracts on cancer: Synergy and xenohormesis. *Medicines* **2018**, *6*, 6. [CrossRef] [PubMed]
22. Barrajon-Catalan, E.; Herranz-Lopez, M.; Joven, J.; Segura-Carretero, A.; Alonso-Villaverde, C.; Menendez, J.A.; Micol, V. Molecular promiscuity of plant polyphenols in the management of age-related diseases: Far beyond their antioxidant properties. *Adv. Exp. Med. Biol.* **2014**, *824*, 141–159. [PubMed]

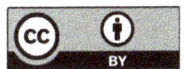

© 2019 by the author. Licensee MDPI, Basel, Switzerland. This article is an open access article distributed under the terms and conditions of the Creative Commons Attribution (CC BY) license (http://creativecommons.org/licenses/by/4.0/).

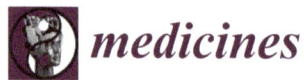

Article

Effect of Sulforaphane and 5-Aza-2′-Deoxycytidine on Melanoma Cell Growth

Tung-chin Chiang [1,*], Brian Koss [2], L. Joseph Su [3], Charity L. Washam [2,4], Stephanie D. Byrum [2,4], Aaron Storey [2] and Alan J. Tackett [2,4,*]

1. Department of Environmental and Occupational Health, University of Arkansas for Medical Sciences, Little Rock, AR 72205, USA
2. Department of Biochemistry & Molecular Biology, University of Arkansas for Medical Sciences, Little Rock, AR 72205, USA
3. Winthrop P. Rockefeller Cancer Institute, Cancer Prevention and Population Sciences Program & Department of Epidemiology, University of Arkansas for Medical Sciences, Little Rock, AR 72205, USA
4. Arkansas Children's Research Institute, Little Rock, AR 72202, USA
* Correspondence: tchiang@uams.edu (T.-c.C.); ajtackett@uams.edu (A.J.T.); Tel.: +1-301-938-6829 (T.-c.C.); +1-501-686-8152 (A.J.T.)

Received: 5 June 2019; Accepted: 24 June 2019; Published: 27 June 2019

Abstract: Background: UV exposure-induced oxidative stress is implicated as a driving mechanism for melanoma. Increased oxidative stress results in DNA damage and epigenetic dysregulation. Accordingly, we explored whether a low dose of the antioxidant sulforaphane (SFN) in combination with the epigenetic drug 5-aza-2′-deoxycytidine (DAC) could slow melanoma cell growth. SFN is a natural bioactivated product of the cruciferous family, while DAC is a DNA methyltransferase inhibitor. **Methods:** Melanoma cell growth characteristics, gene transcription profiles, and histone epigenetic modifications were measured after single and combination treatments with SFN and DAC. **Results:** We detected melanoma cell growth inhibition and specific changes in gene expression profiles upon combinational treatments with SFN and DAC, while no significant alterations in histone epigenetic modifications were observed. Dysregulated gene transcription of a key immunoregulator cytokine—C-C motif ligand 5 (CCL-5)—was validated. **Conclusions:** These results indicate a potential combinatorial effect of a dietary antioxidant and an FDA-approved epigenetic drug in controlling melanoma cell growth.

Keywords: sulforaphane; epigenetic; 5-aza-2′-deoxycytine; melanoma

1. Introduction

While the incidence of certain cancer types has declined, the number of diagnosed melanoma cases has increased sharply over the past three decades [1,2]. Ultraviolet (UV) exposure is one of the most apparent risk factors for melanoma [3]. There are many types of photosensitizers, such as DNA, melanin, and tryptophan, that can receive UV energy and result in direct DNA damage and ROS accumulation [4–6]. UVB affects DNA by forming cyclobutane pyrimidine dimers (CPDs), which lead to DNA mutation [7]. UVA directly induces oxidative stress through the accumulation of 8-oxo-7,8-dihydroguanine (8-oxo-G) and other photoproducts [4]. UV also induces melanin synthesis [8]. There are two types of melanin, eumelanin, and pheomelanin. The ratio of the two types of melanin is dependent on the polymorphism of the melanocortin-1 receptor (MC1R) gene and results in differential pigmentation [6,9]. Synthesis of eumelanin leads to scavenges of reactive oxygen species (ROS) while the synthesis of pheomelanin leads to depletion of antioxidants and results in ROS accumulation [10–12]. This is in concert with the determination that people with pale skin and red hair have low eumelanin and high pheomelanin and are known to have a higher risk of melanoma [13].

Many studies have identified another photosensitizer, tryptophan, which utilizes the energy from UVA and UVB to form a tryptophan photoproduct, 6-formylindolo(3,2-b) carbazole (FICZ) [14,15]. FICZ has a high affinity to the aryl hydrocarbon receptor (AhR) and activates AhR response genes, including cyclooxygenase-2 (Cox2), a melanoma prognostic marker gene [16], and cytochrome P4501A1, which increases ROS accumulation [17]. It has been shown that UVB activates AhR responses that decrease the tumor suppressor gene p27 and impairs nucleotide excision repair (NER) resulting in DNA mutation [18]. In addition to UV exposure, other environmental factors such as cigarette smoking, environmental dioxin 2,3,7,8-tetrachlorodibenzo-p-dioxin (TCDD), and arsenic exposure also induce melanogenesis [3,19–22]. Accumulated ROS from UVA and UVB via different photosensitizers, as well as environmental exposures, have many impacts on cell growth and defense. These impacts include inhibition of p27, cell cycle regulation, increased cytokines, decreased antioxidant glutathione s-transferase, increased 8-oxoG, activation of mitogen-activated protein kinase/extracellular signal-regulated kinases1/2 (MAPK/ERK1/2), increased cell proliferation and decreased tumor suppressor gene p16 [5]. These findings support the fact that melanoma patients have a higher level of oxidative stress and that this stress is associated with the progression of the disease [23].

Studies have shown that environmental exposure-induced DNA damage and oxidative stress can also result in epigenetic changes [24–27]. Elevated ROS is associated with DNA methylation and histone post-translational modifications (PTMs) [25–27]. DNA hypermethylation at promoter CpG sites, especially at tumor suppressor gene promoters, is associated with silencing gene expression in a variety of cancers, including melanoma [28,29]. Many tumor suppressor genes related to cell cycle progression, DNA repair, and apoptosis are methylated in different stages of melanoma [5,24,30–33]. Whole genome DNA methylation profiles from advanced melanoma patients have uncovered a differential methylation pattern that is correlated with survival rates [34]. In addition to aberrant DNA methylation, histone PTMs play critical roles in cancer development independently, in combination with other histone PTMs, and interactively with DNA methylation [24]. Our lab identified the elevation of trimethylation of lysine 27 on histone H3 (H3K27me3) in metastatic melanoma relative to primary melanoma [35]. H3K27me3 is catalyzed by the protein Enhancer of Zeste 2 (EZH2), a member of the Polycomb-group (PcG) family. EZH2 can recruit DNA methyltransferase (DNMT1) to chromatin to form a multisubunit protein complex that suppresses gene expression [36].

Epigenetic therapy using 5-aza-2′-deoxycytidine (DAC), an FDA-approved DNA demethylation agent, has been successfully used to treat myelodysplastic syndromes (MDSs) either alone or in combination with other drugs [37–39]. DAC is a deoxycytidine analog with the replacement of nitrogen at position 5 of the pyrimidine ring [40]. DAC interferes with normal DNA methylation by forming an irreversible covalent bond with DNMT1 [41]. The subsequent DNA-DNMT adducts play a role in controlling cancer cells depending on the dose of DAC. At high doses, DAC induces cytotoxicity by accumulated DNA–DNMT1 adduct-induced apoptosis and DNA synthesis arrest. At low doses, DNA synthesis is continued, while DNA–DNMT1 adduct bonds are being degraded and repaired, resulting in systematically hypomethylated DNA [41,42]. Studies show that DAC has effects on melanoma via decreasing cell growth and invasion [43] as well as alerting gene expression, includes tumor suppressor genes [44].

Regulating oxidative stress via the consumption of antioxidant-rich cruciferous vegetables (e.g., broccoli and Brussels sprouts) has been well-studied in cancer prevention [45–47]. One of the common compounds from cruciferous vegetables with cancer prevention characteristics is glucosinolate. Glucosinolate is not bioactivated until the enzyme myrosinase is released from the plant cell, by chewing or through denaturing by cooking, to catalyze a hydrolytic reaction to form isothiocyanates (ITCs) [48]. Sulforaphane (SFN) is one of the promising anticancer ITCs and can induce biphasic biological impact via generating different level of ROS depending on their doses [48,49]. At a dietary dose, SFN-derived ROS stimulate antioxidant protein expression to balance the ROS level induced from UV exposure. SFN activates nuclear erythroid 2-related factor 2 (Nrf2) to bind to the antioxidant response element at the promoter region of Nrf2-regulated genes. Those genes are phase-II detoxification enzymes (e.g., glutathione S-transferase, quinone reductase, and glucuronosyltransferase). By doing this, SFN increases antioxidant capacity. Furthermore, phase-I enzymes such as P450s, which activate toxic chemical compounds, are reduced by SFN at dietary doses [50–52]. In this way, SFN delivers chemopreventive effects through strengthening cell defense systems by increasing antioxidant enzymes and reducing carcinogen toxicity. Studies have shown that SFN acts as a cell-killing agent at high doses. At a high concentration of SFN, elevated amounts of SFN-derived ROS accumulate in the cells, mitochondrial function is disrupted [49], cell proliferation is blocked, cell cycle G2/M is arrested, and caspase-mediated apoptosis is induced [48,52–55]. High concentrations of SFN also induce epigenetic modification. Studies show that high doses of SFN enhance global histone acetylation by inhibiting histone deacetylase (HDAC) activity and reducing cell growth in prostate cancer [56,57]. The dual roles of SFN in cytoprotection and slowed tumor growth, as well as the low toxicity, are cell-specific [48]. Where and how the ROS is formed by SFN and the impact of surrounding molecular environments has gained great interest in research either with SFN alone or in combination with other chemotherapy drugs in many cancers [58–60].

The research reported here seeks to determine whether combining DAC and SFN can synergistically slow melanoma cell growth. We aimed to utilize a dietary dose of SFN as a natural antioxidant, while at the same time suppressing gene transcription with a low dose of the clinically approved epigenetic modifier DAC. We rationalized that with lower oxidative stress, the low dose of DAC could deliver its epigenetic effect without inducing cytotoxicity. This study is the first step in testing the combined effect of DAC and SFN in a mouse melanoma cell line. Cell growth characteristics, gene expression profiles, and histone PTMs are compared between single and combination treatments of DAC and SFN using mouse melanoma cells. Our data show cell growth inhibition, dysregulation of gene transcription, and increased cytokine production with combination treatment compared to individual treatments. Histone PTMs were identified but did not show differences following treatment. This in-vitro data provides a path to investigate the role of target gene sets and the potential role of the dietary antioxidant SFN in melanoma treatment and prevention.

2. Materials and Methods

2.1. Cell Culture and Treatment

Mouse melanoma B16F10 cells were obtained from ATCC and maintained in Dulbecco's Modified Eagle Medium (DMEM) (ThermoFisher, Waltham, MA, USA) supplemented with 10% FBS (ThermoFisher, Waltham, MA, USA) and 1% penicillin/streptomycin (ThermoFisher, Waltham, MA, USA). Cells were checked for mycoplasma contamination by MycoAler PLUS Mycoplasma Detection Kit (Lonza Walkersville, Walkersville, MD, USA) before experiments.

IC50s for both drugs were determined by using CellTiter 96 AQ$_{ueous}$ One Solution Cell Proliferation Kit (Promega, Madison, WI, USA), following the manufacturer's protocols. In brief, cells were seeded at 1500 cells/well in a 96-well plate for 24 h. Cells were then treated with 5-aza-2′-deoxycytidine (DAC) (Sigma Aldrich, St. Louis, MO, USA) dissolved in dimethyl sulfoxide (DMSO) at concentrations ranging from 25 µM to 6.1 nM (4-fold dilutions from 25 µM, 6.25 µM, 1.56 µM, 390 nM, 97.7 nM, 24.4 nM, to 6.1 nM) for 72 h; and sulforaphane (LKT labs, St Paul, MN, USA) dissolved in water at concentrations ranging from 352 µM to 86 nM (4-fold dilutions ranging from 352 µM, 88.1 µM, 22 µM, 5.5 µM, 1.37 µM, 344 nM, to 86 nM) for 48 h. Dimethyl sulfoxide (DMSO) (Sigma Aldrich, St. Louis, MO, USA) was used as a control in the DMSO wells, at 0.00025%, equivalent to the highest amount of DMSO in the highest dose of treatment (10 mM DAC in DMSO was freshly diluted 400,000 times to 25 nM in culture medium).

Preliminary tests with different doses and duration were performed, based on the results from IC50 measurements, in 6-well plates. The optimal doses and duration of treatments were chosen based on the number of viable cells with greater than 50% of cell survival at single treatment for

DAC and SFN, with fewer cells surviving with combination treatment. SFN at 5 µM and DAC 25 nM were determined to be an optimal dose in the preliminary tests. Cells were seeded in 6-well plates at 4×10^4 cells/well and were allowed to attach for 24 h. For combinatorial drug treatment, cells were treated with DAC at 25 nM for 24 h, the medium was removed, and fresh medium with 25 nM DAC and 5 µM SFN was added. Cells were then incubated for another 48 h. For DAC or SFN single treatment, cells were treated with only DAC or SFN following the same operations as a combination treatment. All treatment groups were harvested at the same time for different target analysis, which included cell number counting and measurements of apoptosis, cell cycle, and gene transcription. Three independent biological repeats were performed.

For cytokine analysis, cells were seeded in 10 cm dishes at 3×10^5 cells/dish and were treated with SFN and DAC as described above in 10% serum-containing medium. Culture medium was replaced from 10% to 1% serum-containing medium with the same dosing scheme at the last 24 h of treatment. The purpose is to reduce potential background. Also, the final culture medium was reduced from 10 mL to 5 mL to increase the concentration of cytokine in the supernatant. The supernatant of each dish was collected for cytokines array analysis. The cell number is calculated to adjust the final amount of supernatant to be loaded from even amount of cells for cytokine analysis.

For CCL5 enzyme-linked immunosorbent assay (ELISA) analysis, cells were grown and treated as described for cytokine array analysis, except the initial cell density is at 2×10^5 cells per 10 cm dish, and the final culture medium was reduced from 10 mL to 5 mL.

For histone analysis, cells were seeded in 10 cm dishes at 2×10^5 cells/dish and were treated with SFN and DAC as described above. Additionally, EZH2 inhibitor EPZ6438 (Med Chem Express, Monmouth Junction, NJ, USA), was used at 5 µM to treat cells for 48 h for analysis of histone epigenetic post-translational modifications. The dose of EPZ6438 was selected for optimal inhibition of the catalytic output of EZH2, histone H3K27me3, and was used as a positive control for histone analysis. DMSO at 0.05%, equivalent to the highest amount of DMSO in the treatment (10 mM EPZ6438 in DMSO was freshly diluted 2000 time to 5 µM in culture medium) was used in the control plates. Three independent biological repeats were performed.

2.2. Assays for Characteristics of Cell Growth

2.2.1. Viable Cell Count

Cell number was counted with Trypan blue solution (0.4%) using a hemocytometer. The number of the cell count was controlled to within 20–50 cells/square via dilution of cells before mixing with trypan blue.

2.2.2. Cell Cycle Arrest Analysis

Cells cycle was analyzed by fixing cells in 70% ethanol overnight and staining with propidium iodide (PI)/RNase Staining Buffer (BD Biosciences, San Jose, CA, USA). The stained DNA was analyzed at the University of Arkansas for Medical Sciences (UAMS) flow cytometry core with an LSRFortessa Flow cytometer (BD Biosciences, San Jose, CA, USA). Flow cytometry data were analyzed with Flow Jo (Ashland, OR, USA) and Dean-Jett Fox (DJF) model (BD, Franklin Lakes, NJ, USA).

2.2.3. Apoptotic Analysis

Apoptosis was measured by Annexin V and 4′,6-diamidino-2-phenylindole (DAPI) staining using the annexin V-FITC apoptosis detection kit (BD Pharmigen, San Jose, CA, USA), following the manufacturer's protocol. Cells were analyzed at the UAMS flow cytometry core with an LSRFortessa Flow cytometer (BD Biosciences, San Jose, CA, USA). Flow cytometry data were analyzed with Flow Jo (Ashland, OR, USA).

2.3. RNA-Seq Analysis

2.3.1. RNA Extraction and Targeted Gene Expression Analysis

RNA was extracted with the RNeasy Mini Kit (Qiagen, Germantown, MD, USA) following the manufacturer's protocols and eluted in water. RNA was reversed transcribed into cDNA with the One Step iScript kit (BioRad, Hercules, CA, USA) following the manufacturer's protocol.

Targeted genes of interest were amplified with 20 ng of cDNA, SYBR green Supermix (Bio-Rad, Hercules, CA, USA) and primers (final concentration at 750 nM). The PCR cyclic conditions used were 95 °C for 3 min, followed by 39 cycles of 98 °C for 15 s and 57 °C for 30 s. The following primer pairs (Integrated DNA Technologies, Coralville, IA, USA) were used for real-time analysis (Table 1):

Table 1. Primers.

Ccl5-Forward	ACCATATGGCTCGGACACCA
Ccl5-Reverse	TCTCTGGGTTGGCACACACTT
IL33-Forward	GGGGCTCACTGCAGGAAAGT
IL33-Reverse	ATTTTGCAAGGCGGGACCAG
Dusp15-Forward	TATCCACGAATCACCCCA
Dusp15-Reverse	AAGCAGTGCACAAGGCA
UBC-forward	GCCCAGTGTTACCACCAAGAGCC
UBC-Reverse	CCCATCACACCCAAGAACAGTT

Ccl5: (C-C motif) ligand 5 (Gene ID:20304); IL33: interleukin 33 (Gene ID:77125); Dusp15: dual specificity phosphatase-like 15 (Gene ID:252864); UBC: Ubiquitin C (Gene ID: 22190).

2.3.2. RNA-Seq Sample Preparation

cDNA libraries were constructed using Illumina's TruSeq stranded mRNA sample preparation kit according to the manufacturer's protocol. Briefly, 500 ng of total RNA was polyA selected, chemically fragmented, and converted to single-stranded cDNA using random hexamer-primed reverse transcription. Second strand synthesis was then performed to generate double-stranded cDNA, followed by fragment end repair and the addition of a single A base to each end of the cDNA. Adapters, including a 3' adapter and a 5' adapter containing 1 of 48 unique indexes, were then ligated to the fragment ends to enable attachment to the sequencing flow cell and sample pooling. Next, library DNA was PCR amplified and validated for fragment size and quantity using an Advanced Analytical Fragment Analyzer (AATI) and Qubit fluorometer (Life Technologies), respectively. Equal amounts (5 µL of 4 nM dilutions) of each library were pooled and 5 µL of the pool was denatured for 5 min by the addition of 5 µL of 0.2 N NaOH, incubated at room temperature for 5 min, neutralized by the addition of 5 µL 200 mM Tris pH 7.0, and diluted to a loading concentration of 1.8 pM; 1.3 mL of the denatured, diluted library was added to a NextSeq reagent cartridge V2.0 for sequencing on a NextSeq 500 platform using a high output flow cell to generate approximately 25 million 75-base reads per sample. All sequencing was conducted by the Center for Translational Pediatric Research Genomics Core Lab at Arkansas Children's Research Institute (Little Rock, AR, USA).

2.3.3. RNA-Seq Data Analysis

RNA reads were checked for quality of sequencing using FastQC v.0.11.7 (http://www.bioinformatics.babraham.ac.uk/projects/fastqc/). The adaptors and low-quality bases (Q < 20) were trimmed to a minimum of 36 base pairs using Trimmomatic v0.38 [61]. Reads that passed quality control were aligned to the mouse (mm10) (GCA_000001305.2) reference genome using TopHat v2.1.1 [62]. Sample alignment files (.bam) were then imported into Blast2GO v5.1.13, and gene level expression counts quantified using htseq [63,64]. Only reads uniquely aligned to known genes were retained and counted. Multimapped reads were discarded. Genes with low counts were then removed before downstream analysis. To retain the maximum number of interesting features genes with a minimum of 1 counts-per-million (CPM) values in at least 3 libraries were retained for further investigation. The filtered dataset was then normalized for compositional bias using a trimmed mean of M values (TMM) and $\log_2$ transformed [65]. For each comparison, edgeR quasi-likelihood method (glmQLFTest) correcting for batch effect was used to identify differentially expressed genes between experimental groups [2]. Genes with multiple tests corrected (FDR) p-values of 0.05 [66] and a fold change > 2 were selected for further comparisons between treatments and analyzed by Ingenuity Pathway Analysis (IPA) for biological involvement.

2.4. Chemokines Analysis

The supernatant of control and combination treated groups was spun at 10,000 g for 5 min to remove the cell debris. The supernatant was added to the membrane of Proteome Profiler mouse XL Cytokine array kit (R&D system Inc, Minneapolis, MN, USA). The manufactural protocol was followed with modification at the final film developing. Western Lightning Plus-ECL (PerkinElmer, Waltham, MA, USA) was applied at the end of film developing to have clear signals.

For ELISA, the supernatant was spun at 10,000 g for 5 min to remove the cell debris and further diluted 10 times in 1 × PBS. Duplicate diluted supernatant from each group and the serially diluted standards (ranging from 7.8 pg/mL to 500 pg/mL) were tested for the level of CCL5 according to the manufacturer's instructions (R&D Systems Inc., Minneapolis, MN, USA). The cell number is also calculated and applied in data analysis to reflect the level of CCL5 in the supernatant is from the same amount of cells.

2.5. Histone PTM Mass Spectrometry

Histones were purified from approximately 5 million cells by acid extraction, as described by Taverna, SD et al. [67]. The amount of protein was quantified by BCA Protein Assay Kit (ThermoFisher, Waltham, MA, USA). Extracted histones (5 μg), were resolved on a 4–20% gradient SDS-PAGE gel. Histone bands were visualized by staining with GelCode Blue (Thermo). Histones were excised from the gel, destained, and treated with 20 μL/band of 30% d6-acetic anhydride in 50 mM ammonium bicarbonate. Histones were then digested in-gel with 125 ng/band sequencing-grade trypsin at 37 °C overnight. Acidified tryptic peptides were separated using a 2.5 μm Waters XSelect CSH resin on a 150 mm × 0.075 mm column using a nanoAcquity UPLC system (Waters, Milford, MA, USA). Peptides were separated using a 60-min chromatography gradient, with a 40-min linear separation gradient from 97% buffer A (0.1% formic acid in water (v/v)), 3% buffer B (0.1% formic acid (v/v), 99.9% acetonitrile (v/v)), to 80% of buffer A, 20% buffer B. Eluted peptides were ionized by electrospray (2150 V) and analyzed on an Orbitrap Fusion Lumos mass spectrometer (Thermo Fisher, Waltham, MA, USA) using data-dependent acquisition. A full-scan MS was acquired in profile mode at 120,000 resolution from 375 to 1500 m/z (AGC target 5×10^5, max injection time 100 ms), followed by data-dependent MS/MS analysis with a 3 second duty cycle time. Peptides with a determined monoisotopic peak, intensity threshold greater than 2×10^4 counts, and charge state of 2–7 were selected for HCD fragmentation at 30% collision energy, AGC target of 1×10^4, maximum injection time 35 milliseconds, and analyzed in the ion trap with scan speed set to rapid.

Raw data files were analyzed using Mascot (Matrix Science, London, UK) using a custom Uniprot database which included only mouse histones (Table 2). Files were searched with a precursor tolerance of 3 ppm and fragment ion tolerance of 0.5 Da. Fixed modifications included carbamidomethylation of cysteine. Variable modifications to lysine included monomethylation, dimethylation, trimethylation, acetylation, deuterated acetylation, and methylation and deuterated acetylation. Variable modifications to arginine included monomethylation and dimethylation. Variable modifications to serine and threonine were phosphorylation. Up to four missed trypsin cleavages were permitted. Mascot search results were loaded into Scaffold, and filtered for a protein FDR of 1%, a peptide score probability of

80%, and a minimum of 5 peptides per protein. Spectral count data was exported in tabular format and analyzed using R [68].

Table 2. List of mouse histones used for analysis.

Mouse Histones					
H10	H1FOO	H2A2B	H2AX	H2B1H	H2B3B
H11	H1T	H2A2C	H2AY	H2B1K	H31
H12	H2A1	H2A3	H2AZ	H2B1M	H32
H13	H2A1F	H2AB1	H2B1A	H2B1P	H33
H14	H2A1H	H2AJ	H2B1B	H2B2B	H3C
H15	H2A1K	H2AV	H2B1C	H2B2E	H4
H1FNT	H2A2A	H2AW	H2B1F	H2B3A	

3. Results

3.1. SFN and DAC Single and Combination Treatment Result in Growth Inhibition

The IC50 for SFN was calculated to be approximately 22 µM for SFN and 44 nM for DAC (Figure 1A). For cell growth inhibition, a dose of 5 µM of SFN and 25 nM of DAC were chosen based on cell viability assays with more than 50% cells surviving from a single treatment of SFN and DAC respectively. Viable cell counts were calculated in the single and combination treatment of DAC and SFN compared to control (Figure 1B). There was 58% ± 4% and 56% ± 7% viable cells compared to control for the single treatment with DAC and SFN, respectively and only 33% ± 5% of viable cells in SFN and DAC combination treatment. The combination treatment induced significant growth inhibition compared to any single treatment ($p < 0.03$, Student's t-test).

3.2. SFN and DAC Single and Combination Treatment Result in Minimal Apoptosis

Apoptosis analysis showed that most of the cells were noted as alive by negative stain for annexin V and DAPI in all treatments and control (Figure 1C,D). The percentage of viable cells not in apoptosis with DAC and SFN single treatments, was 99% ± 0.2% ($p < 0.01$) and 97% ± 1% ($p < 0.01$), respectively, compared to control. Combination treatment of DAC and SFN results in 95% ± 1% ($p < 0.004$) of viable cells compared to control. The percentage of viable cells not in apoptosis with combination treatments was slightly lower than any single treatment of SFN ($p < 0.03$) and DAC ($p < 0.01$).

3.3. SFN and DAC Single and Combination Treatment Result in No Cell Cycle Arrest

Cell cycle analysis indicated that all treated and control cells were in normal distributions for different cell cycles with G1 as dominant, followed by S phase and G2 phase, as shown in representative figures (Figure 1E). There was no significant difference between treatments in the G2/M phase (Figure 1F).

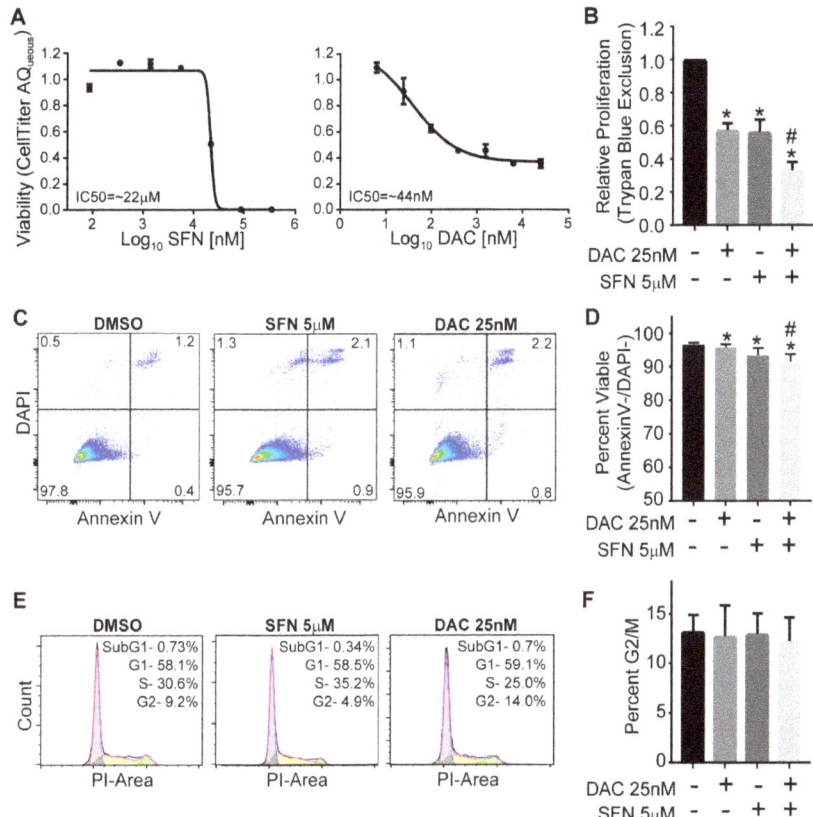

Figure 1. Impact of SFN and DAC single and combination treatment on the growth of B16 melanoma. (**A**) The IC50 of SFN and DAC single treatment is approximately 22 µM and 44 nM, respectively. Cell viability was determined using the CellTiter 96 AQ$_\text{ueous}$ One Solution Cell Proliferation kit. The data were analyzed by nonlinear regression to determine the IC50. (**B**) Growth inhibition induced from single and combination treatment of SFN and DAC. Viable cells were measured by trypan blue staining and analyzed by Student's t-test. (**C**) Representative apoptosis analysis (AnnexinV/DAPI) by flow cytometry from control, SFN, and DAC single treatment. (**D**) The percentage of viable cells with DAC and SFN single and combination treatments were compared to control. (**E**) Representative cell cycle analysis from control and SFN and DAC single treatment. Data were analyzed with Flow Jo /Dean-Jett Fox (DJF) model. (**F**) The percent G2/M phase in DAC and SFN single and combination treatments were compared to control with Student's t-test. * Significantly different from control, # Single treatment is significantly different from combinational treatment (Student's t-test).

3.4. SFN Induced Dysregulated Gene Transcription

RNAseq data analysis revealed a differential gene expression profile by SFN single treatment compared to control. There were 126 genes with greater than 2-fold change compared to control. The data have been deposited in NCBI's Gene Expression Omnibus [69]. The top genes with greater than 2.5-fold change ($p < 0.001$) are shown in the heatmap (Figure 2A). The biological roles of genes responding to SFN single treatment with greater than 2-fold change were analyzed with IPA. The top canonical pathways analysis, with a negative log p-value greater than 2, indicated many important biological pathways dysregulated in response to SFN single treatment (Figure 2B).

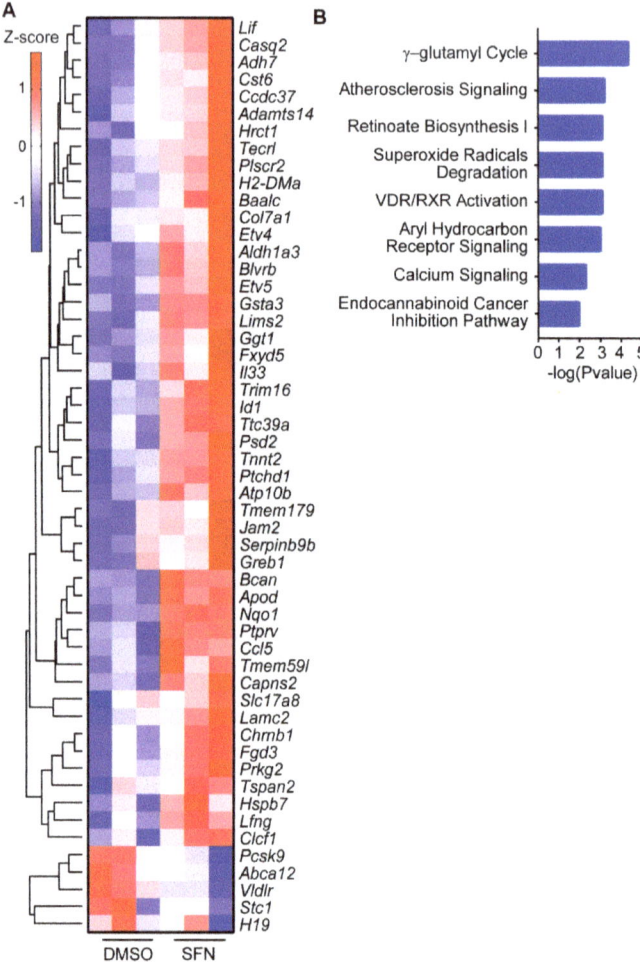

Figure 2. Differential gene expression induced by SFN single treatment and the related biological pathways. (**A**) Differentially expressed genes from SFN single treatment compared to control. Genes with greater than 2.5 fold changes ($p < 0.001$) were analyzed with unsupervised clustering (Z score shown in the color key). (**B**) Top canonical pathways from SFN single treatment. Genes greater than two-fold change relative to control were analyzed with Ingenuity Pathway Analysis (IPA) for their biological significance. The top eight pathways are shown here.

3.5. SFN and DAC Uniquely Induced Dysregulated Gene Transcription

DAC single treatment induced 19 genes to greater than 2-fold change compared to control ($p < 0.05$), and this number is too low for canonical pathway analysis by IPA. However, SFN and DAC combination treatment induced more genes than any single treatment. There were 261 genes with greater than a 2-fold change from the combination treatment of SFN and DAC compared to control ($p < 0.05$). The data from DAC single and SFN and DAC combination treatment have been deposited in NCBI's Gene Expression Omnibus [69] as described above for SFN single treatment with the same accession number GSE12752. The top genes with greater than 3-fold change ($p < 0.001$) induced from SFN and DAC combination treatment are shown in the heatmap (Figure 3A). The biological roles of genes responded to SFN and DAC combination treatment compared to control with greater than 2-fold change were analyzed with IPA. The top canonical pathways analysis, with a negative log *p*-value greater than 3.5, showed many biological pathways involvement (Figure 3B). The role of vitamin D receptor/retinoid X receptor (VDR/RXR) activation and aryl hydrocarbon receptor signaling were listed as the top two canonical pathways from SFN and DAC combination treatment with a negative log *p*-value greater than 5.5. These two pathways were also detected in SFN single treatment with a negative log *p*-value approximately 3.0 (Figure 2B).

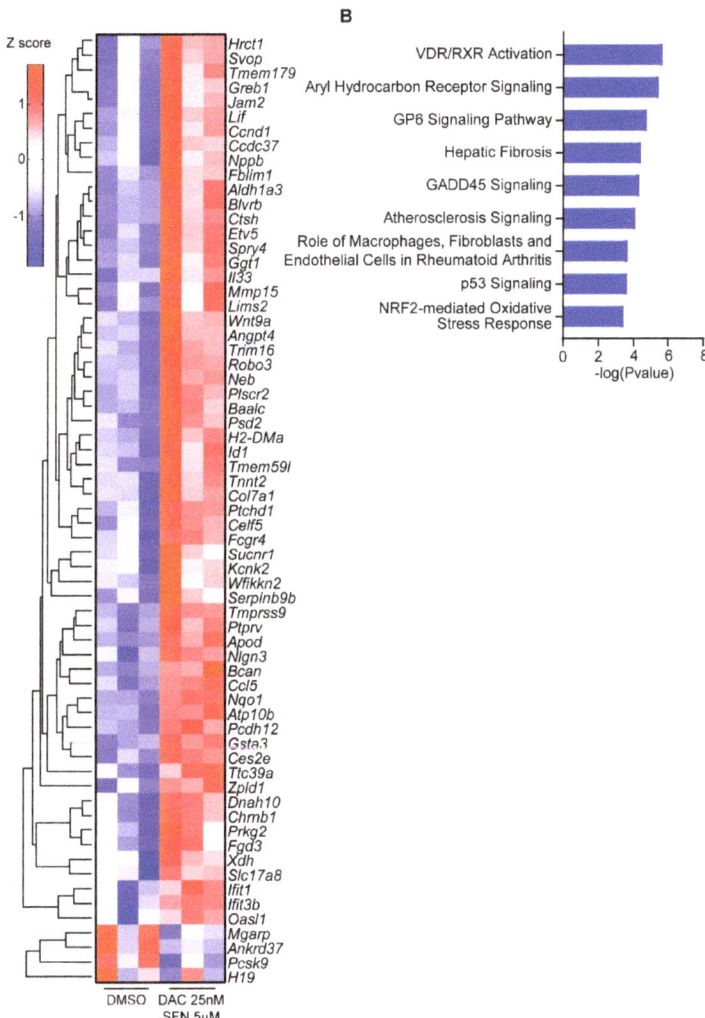

Figure 3. Differential gene expression induced by SFN and DAC combination treatment and the involved biological pathways. (**A**) Differentially expressed genes from the combination treatment of SFN and DAC compared to control treatments. Genes with greater than 3-fold change ($p < 0.001$) were analyzed with unsupervised clustering (Z score shown in the color key). (**B**) Top canonical pathways from the combination treatment of SFN and DAC. Genes greater than 2-fold change than the control with the combination treatment of SFN and DAC were analyzed with IPA for their biological significance. The top nine pathways are shown here.

3.6. Validation of Dysregulated Gene Transcription Induced by SFN and DAC Combination Treatment

There were 261 genes with greater than 2-fold change ($p < 0.05$) of gene expression (either increased or decreased) with DAC plus SFN combination treatments compared to control. The number of genes with expression changes greater than 2-fold ($p < 0.05$), compared to control, from the single treatment were 19 and 126 genes for DAC and SFN, respectively (Figure 4A). Furthermore, there were 150 unique genes from combination treatment compared to control (Figure 4B).

We selected genes for further validation from the SFN and DAC combination treatment with greater than 2-fold change compared to control. The preliminary selection criteria from RNA-seq data were genes with the highest differential expression compared to control or involved in multiple top biological pathways (Figure 4C). Three genes, CCL5, DUSP15, and IL33, were validated by reverse transcription PCR (RT-PCR) (Figure 4D). These genes were selected for validation on the criteria that they showed differential expression between single treatment and control as well as between combination treatment and single treatment. CCL5 increased 2 ± 0.1 ($p < 2.4 \times 10^{-6}$) and 3 ± 0.2 ($p < 1.5 \times 10^{-5}$) times with single treatment of DAC and SFN, respectively, and increased 5 ± 0.2 ($p < 1.3 \times 10^{-7}$, Student's t-test) with combination treatment compared to control. DUSP15 increased 1.7 ± 0.2 ($p < 6.2 \times 10^{-3}$) and 1.9 ± 0.1 ($p < 8.7 \times 10^{-6}$) times with single treatment of DAC and SFN, respectively, and increased 3.6 ± 0.3 ($p < 1.7 \times 10^{-5}$, Student's t-test) with combination treatment compared to control. IL33 increased 1.6 ± 0.3 ($p < 4.2 \times 10^{-2}$) and 2.2 ± 0.2 ($p < 2.0 \times 10^{-4}$) times with single treatment of DAC and SFN, respectively, and increased 3.0 ± 0.3 ($p < 2.1 \times 10^{-4}$, Student's t-test) with combination treatment compared to control.

The level of secreted cytokines CCL5 and IL33, as well as other 111 cytokines, were measured in the supernatant using a mouse XL cytokines array (Figure 4E). Out of the 111 mouse cytokines probes on the membrane, CCL5 was detected with greater than two times increased signal in combination treatment compared to the control group. IL33 was not present at detectable levels. Other cytokines, such as CXCL10 (Gene ID 15945), angiopoietin-2 (Gene ID 11601), CD105 (Gene ID 13805), VEGF (Gene ID 22339), and CCN4 (Gene ID 22402), were detected with an increased level of expression in combination treatment than control.

Specific CCL5 ELISA further confirmed the increase in CCL 5 in DAC/SFN combination treatment, as indicated in Figure 4F. The level of CCL5 in control is about 55 +/− 22.3 pg/mL and is increased to 348 +/− 92.2 pg/mL in SFN/DAC combination treatment from two independent biological runs.

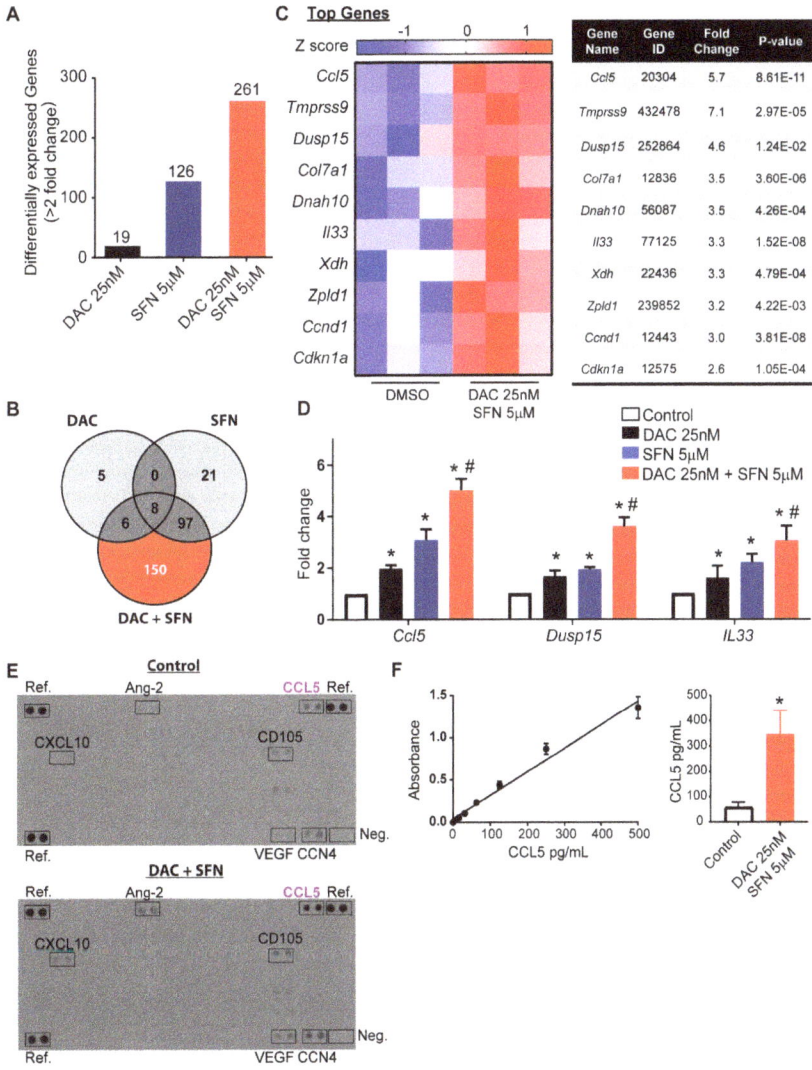

Figure 4. Validation of combination effects from SFN and DAC. (**A**) The number of differentially expressed genes induced by different treatments. (**B**) The number of unique genes responding to single and combination treatment. All genes were selected from greater than 2-fold change compared to control with $p < 0.05$. (**C**) A heatmap and list of top selected genes from SFN and DAC combination treatments (Z score shows in the color key). (**D**) Relative gene expression validation by rtPCR of Ccl5, Dusp15, and IL33 between treatments. * Significantly different from control, $p < 0.05$, # Single treatment is significantly different from combinational treatment, $p < 0.05$ (Student's *t*-test). (**E**) Expression of cytokines detected by cytokine array. Ref indicates reference spots. Neg: negative control. Arrays were performed in duplicate. (**F**) Specific CCL5 ELISA further confirmed the increase in CCL 5 in DAC/SFN combination treatment. The left side indicated the standard curve of CCL5, ranged from 7.8 pg/mL to 500 pg/mL. The right side indicates the concentration of CCL5 in the supernatant is increased from 55pg/mL in control to 348 pg/mL in DAC/SFN combination treated group. All data were from two independent biological runs.

3.7. Analysis of Histone Epigenetic Post-Translational Modifications (PTMs)

Post-translational modifications were identified and subsequently quantified on histones H3 and H4. EPZ treatment is known to decrease H3K27me3, and was consequently used as a positive control. We treated cells with EPZ6438 for 48 hrs along with SFN and DAC combination treatments as described in the methods section. Histone PTMs were analyzed using lysine derivatization and a bottom-up proteomic workflow. Aside from positive control, no significant differences in histone PTMs were detected (Supplementary Figure S1).

4. Discussion

For the current study, we explored the possibility of controlling melanoma cell growth by combining the antioxidant SFN and the epigenetic drug DAC. The rationale behind this work was to control the level of ROS while altering the epigenetic status with a relatively low dose of each drug. The aim is to lay the first step for our long term goal in using a dietary dose of an antioxidant to help epigenetic drugs in controlling melanoma. Therefore, we aimed to use a low dose of each drug to allow the future application of a dietary dose of SFN and a low dose of DAC to reduce side effects. We chose 5 µM of SFN and 25 nM of DAC, which are equal to or lower than half of the respective IC50 from our test (Figure 1A). These doses of the drugs induce significant growth inhibition with combination treatment compared to control and either single treatment (Figure 1B). We did not find apoptosis or cell cycle arrest in any treatments (Figure 1C–F). This finding is different from other studies using a higher dose of each drug (6–25 µM of SFN [70,71] and 200 nM–0.5 µM of DAC [72,73]). These higher-dose studies all demonstrate apoptosis and cell arrest effects. At the low doses used in this study, the two drugs induced different mechanisms as compared to studies using relatively high doses of SFN or DAC. Our findings suggest that the growth inhibition may be involved in mechanisms other than apoptosis and cell cycle arrest. A combination treatment of low-dose SFN and DAC reduced the cell growth without initiating cell cycle arrest or apoptosis. These data indicate that attenuating ROS with the antioxidant SFN may enhance the utility of the epigenetic drug DAC in controlling cell growth, with less impact on the host.

We investigated the impact of this drug combination at the transcriptional level by RNAseq (Figures 2 and 3). There was a significant increase in the total number of genes with greater than 2-fold ($p < 0.05$) expression change in cells that received the combination treatment as compared to those that received either single treatment and as compared to control (Figure 4A). The absolute number of genes altered by 25 nM of DAC is very low at 19, and those altered by SFN alone is higher at 126. This may be attributed to the low dose treatment with limited impact. Interestingly, the number of altered genes increased to 261 when SFN and DAC combination treatment was applied. The top differentially-expressed genes and canonical pathways showed different distributions between single SFN and combination SFN and DAC treatment (Figures 2 and 3). VDR/RXR activation and aryl hydrocarbon receptor signaling (AhR receptor) are two top-listed pathways from combination treatments. Both pathways are known to be associated with UV exposure [5,15,74–76]. We validated select genes involved in more than one canonical pathway or listed as top differentially-expressed genes (Figure 4C). The transcription level of the three genes (CCL5, IL33, and DUSP15) were significantly higher in the combination treatment than either of the single treatments (Figure 4D). Two (CCL5 and IL33) of the three genes are secreted proteins. We further validated secreted proteins with cytokine arrays and ELISA on CCL5 (Figure 4E,F). CCL5 was validated to have increased levels, both in transcription level and detected extracellularly after combination treatment as compared to control. CCL5 is also known as RANTES (regulated on activation, normal T cell expressed and secreted). It is one of the cytokines which functions as a chemoattractant for natural killer (NK) cells [77], which do not efficiently infiltrate solid tumors such as melanoma [78]. CCL5 is the main factor in inhibiting melanoma growth by bringing NK cells to the tumor site, while autophagy is suppressed [79]. Activated NK cells could stimulate the immune checkpoint programmed cell death protein 1 (PD-1) [80] and cytotoxic T lymphocytes (CTL)-associated antigen 4 (CTLA4) [81] to deliver immunoregulatory effects. Increased expression of CCL5 involves the phosphorylation of the MAPK8/JNK-JUN/c-Jun signaling pathway, which is initiated by decreased expression of protein phosphatase 2 A (PP2A), while autophagy is suppressed [82,83]. Clinically, a high level of CCL5 is positively associated with the NK cell marker NKp46 as well as with melanoma patients' survival [79,84].

We also investigated whether low dose treatments of SFN and DAC have an impact on histone PTMs. There was no differential PTMs detected when control and combination of SNF and DAC treated cells were analyzed (Supplementary Figure S1). This suggests that under the conditions of our treatments, the differential gene expression and cell inhibition may not be associated with histone epigenetic reprogramming, but rather the direct effects of SFN and DAC.

In summary, our data suggest that attenuating ROS through the use of the antioxidant SFN can help the epigenetic drug DAC control cell growth. This control is not via direct cell killing with apoptosis, cell cycle arrest or histone modifications, but, more directly, by changing gene transcription and cytokine production, which may increase the immune defense system by recruiting natural killer cells.

5. Conclusions

Melanoma patients not only have high oxidative stress [23], but also have a high frequency of recurrence of the disease [85,86]. It is apparent that melanoma patients are susceptible to daily UV- and environmental exposure-induced ROS [5]. Managing the level of ROS via natural antioxidants has demonstrated beneficial effects in controlling melanoma [5], but does not eliminate the tumor. Our study aimed to attenuate ROS by a low dose of the antioxidant SFN and allow the epigenetic drug DAC to control melanoma at a lower dose. The current study clearly demonstrates that SFN could have combinational effects with the commonly used, FDA-approved demethylation agent DAC in significantly inhibiting melanoma cell growth. The next goal is to apply our findings to animal studies. The long term goal is for the clinical application of controlling melanoma with a dietary dose of SFN and target drugs (e.g., epigenetic and immunotherapeutic drugs) at lower doses that may have fewer side effects for patients.

Supplementary Materials: The following are available online at http://www.mdpi.com/2305-6320/6/3/71/s1, Figure S1: Histone post-translational modifications on Histone H3 (A) and H4 (B) were detected upon EPZ6438 treatment as well as SFN and DAC combination treatment. As anticipated for the positive control, H3K27me3 was significantly lower following EPZ treatment.

Author Contributions: Conceptualization: T.-c.C., L.J.S., and A.J.T.; Methodology: T.-c.C., B.K., L.J.S., C.L.W., S.D.B., A.S., and A.J.T.; Formal analysis: T.-c.C., B.K., C.L.W., and S.D.B.; Resources: L.J.S. and A.J.T. Data curation: T.-c.C., C.L.W., A.S., and B.K.; Writing; T.-c.C., B.K., S.D.B., A.S., L.J.S., and A.J.T.; Visualization: B.K.; Supervision: T.-c.C., L.J.S., and A.J.T.; Project administration: T.-c.C. and A.J.T; Funding acquisition: L.J.S. and A.J.T.

Funding: We acknowledge support from NIH grant P20GM121293, NIH grant R01CA236209, and the Scharlau Family Endowed Chair in Cancer Research to AJT. This study was additionally supported by the National Institutes of Health (UL1TR000039, P20GM103625, S10OD018445, and P20GM103429).

Acknowledgments: Rosalind B Penny for critical editing and review; Hui-Yi Lin for data analysis consultation; Jun Nakamura for idea generation and critical review; Winthrop P. Rockefeller Cancer Institute, University of Arkansas for Medical Science; Department of Biochemistry and Molecular Biology, University of Arkansas for Medical Science; and the Chancellor's Challenge Initiative of the University of Arkansas: Global Expression Pathway Analysis Training: Target Obesity.

Conflicts of Interest: The authors declare no conflicts of interest.

References

1. Sandru, A.; Voinea, S.; Panaitescu, E.; Blidaru, A. Survival rates of patients with metastatic malignant melanoma. *J. Med. Life* **2014**, *7*, 572–576. [PubMed]
2. Chen, Y.; Lun, A.T.; Smyth, G.K. From reads to genes to pathways: Differential expression analysis of RNA-Seq experiments using Rsubread and the edgeR quasi-likelihood pipeline. *F1000Research* **2016**, *5*, 1438. [PubMed]
3. Berwick, M.; Buller, D.B.; Cust, A.; Gallagher, R.; Lee, T.K.; Meyskens, F.; Pandey, S.; Thomas, N.E.; Veierød, M.B.; Ward, S. Melanoma Epidemiology and Prevention. *Cancer Treat. Res.* **2016**, *167*, 17–49. [PubMed]

4. Cadet, J.; Wagner, J.R. DNA base damage by reactive oxygen species, oxidizing agents, and UV radiation. *Cold Spring Harb. Perspect. Biol.* **2013**, *5*, a012559. [CrossRef] [PubMed]
5. Venza, M.; Visalli, M.; Beninati, C.; Gaetano, G.V.D.; Teti, D.; Venza, I. Cellular Mechanisms of Oxidative Stress and Action in Melanoma. *Oxid. Med. Cell. Longev.* **2015**, *2015*, 1–11. [CrossRef] [PubMed]
6. Videira, I.F.; Moura, D.F.; Magina, S. Mechanisms regulating melanogenesis. *Bras. Derm.* **2013**, *88*, 76–83. [CrossRef] [PubMed]
7. Drouin, R.; Therrien, J.P. UVB-induced cyclobutane pyrimidine dimer frequency correlates with skin cancer mutational hotspots in p53. *Photochem. Photobiol.* **1997**, *66*, 719–726. [CrossRef]
8. Abdel-Malek, Z.; Swope, V.; Smalara, D.; Babcock, G.; Dawes, S.; Nordlund, J. Analysis of the UV-induced melanogenesis and growth arrest of human melanocytes. *Pigment Cell Res.* **1994**, *7*, 326–332. [CrossRef]
9. Latreille, J.; Ezzedine, K.; Elfakir, A.; Ambroisine, L.; Gardinier, S.; Galan, P.; Hercberg, S.; Gruber, G.; Rees, J.; Tschachler, E.; et al. MC1R gene polymorphism affects skin color and phenotypic features related to sun sensitivity in a population of French adult women. *Photochem. Photobiol.* **2009**, *85*, 1451–1458. [CrossRef]
10. Morgan, A.M.; Lo, J.; Fisher, D.E. How does pheomelanin synthesis contribute to melanomagenesis?: Two distinct mechanisms could explain the carcinogenicity of pheomelanin synthesis. *Bioessays* **2013**, *35*, 672–676. [CrossRef]
11. Hsiao, J.J.; Fisher, D.E. The roles of microphthalmia-associated transcription factor and pigmentation in melanoma. *Arch. Biochem. Biophys.* **2014**, *563*, 28–34. [CrossRef] [PubMed]
12. Samokhvalov, A.; Hong, L.; Liu, Y.; Garguilo, J.; Nemanich, R.J.; Edwards, G.S.; Simon, J.D. Oxidation potentials of human eumelanosomes and pheomelanosomes. *Photochem. Photobiol.* **2005**, *81*, 145–148. [CrossRef] [PubMed]
13. Sulem, P.; Gudbjartsson, D.F.; Stacey, S.N.; Helgason, A.; Rafnar, T.; Magnusson, K.P.; Manolescu, A.; Karason, A.; Palsson, A.; Thorleifsson, G.; et al. Genetic determinants of hair, eye and skin pigmentation in Europeans. *Nat. Genet.* **2007**, *39*, 1443–1452. [CrossRef] [PubMed]
14. Syed, D.N.; Mukhtar, H. FICZ: A Messenger of Light in Human Skin. *J. Investig. Derm.* **2015**, *135*, 1478–1481. [CrossRef] [PubMed]
15. Fritsche, E.; Schäfer, C.; Calles, C.; Bernsmann, T.; Bernshausen, T.; Wurm, M.; Hübenthal, U.; Cline, J.E.; Hajimiragha, H.; Schroeder, P.; et al. Lightening up the UV response by identification of the arylhydrocarbon receptor as a cytoplasmatic target for ultraviolet B radiation. *Proc. Natl. Acad. Sci. USA* **2007**, *104*, 8851–8856. [CrossRef] [PubMed]
16. Becker, M.R.; Siegelin, M.D.; Rompel, R.; Enk, A.H.; Gaiser, T. COX-2 expression in malignant melanoma: A novel prognostic marker? *Melanoma Res.* **2009**, *19*, 8–16. [CrossRef] [PubMed]
17. Furue, M.; Takahara, M.; Nakahara, T.; Uchi, H. Role of AhR/ARNT system in skin homeostasis. *Arch. Derm. Res.* **2014**, *306*, 769–779. [CrossRef] [PubMed]
18. Pollet, M.; Shaik, S.; Mescher, M.; Frauenstein, K.; Tigges, J.; Braun, S.A.; Sondenheimer, K.; Kaveh, M.; Bruhs, A.; Meller, S.; et al. The AHR represses nucleotide excision repair and apoptosis and contributes to UV-induced skin carcinogenesis. *Cell Death Differ.* **2018**, *25*, 1823–1836. [CrossRef]
19. Delijewski, M.; Wrześniok, D.; Otręba, M.; Beberok, A.; Rok, J.; Buszman, E. Nicotine impact on melanogenesis and antioxidant defense system in HEMn-DP melanocytes. *Mol. Cell. Biochem.* **2014**, *395*, 109–116. [CrossRef]
20. Haresaku, S.; Hanioka, T.; Tsutsui, A.; Watanabe, T. Association of lip pigmentation with smoking and gingival melanin pigmentation. *Oral Dis.* **2007**, *13*, 71–76. [CrossRef]
21. Mimura, J.; Fujii-Kuriyama, Y. Functional role of AhR in the expression of toxic effects by TCDD. *Biochim. Biophys. Acta* **2003**, *1619*, 263–268. [CrossRef]
22. Granstein, R.D.; Sober, A.J. Drug- and heavy metal—Induced hyperpigmentation. *J. Am. Acad. Derm.* **1981**, *5*, 1–18. [CrossRef]
23. Bisevac, J.P.; Djukic, M.; Stanojevic, I.; Stevanovic, I.; Mijuskovic, Z.; Djuric, A.; Gobeljic, B.; Banovic, T.; Vojvodic, D. Association Between Oxidative Stress and Melanoma Progression. *J. Med. Biochem.* **2018**, *37*, 12–20. [CrossRef] [PubMed]
24. Sarkar, D.; Leung, E.Y.; Baguley, B.C.; Finlay, G.J.; Askarian-Amiri, M.E. Epigenetic regulation in human melanoma: Past and future. *Epigenetics* **2015**, *10*, 103–121. [CrossRef] [PubMed]
25. Tokarz, P.; Kaarniranta, K.; Blasiak, J. Inhibition of DNA methyltransferase or histone deacetylase protects retinal pigment epithelial cells from DNA damage induced by oxidative stress by the stimulation of antioxidant enzymes. *Eur. J. Pharm.* **2016**, *776*, 167–175. [CrossRef] [PubMed]

26. Donkena, K.V.; Young, C.Y.; Tindall, D.J. Oxidative stress and DNA methylation in prostate cancer. *Obs. Gynecol. Int.* **2010**, *2010*, 1–14. [CrossRef]
27. Wachsman, J.T. DNA methylation and the association between genetic and epigenetic changes: Relation to carcinogenesis. *Mutat. Res.* **1997**, *375*, 1–8. [CrossRef]
28. Sigalotti, L.; Covre, A.; Fratta, E.; Parisi, G.; Colizzi, F.; Rizzo, A.; Danielli, R.; Nicolay, H.J.; Coral, S.; Maio, M. Epigenetics of human cutaneous melanoma: Setting the stage for new therapeutic strategies. *J. Transl. Med.* **2010**, *8*, 56. [CrossRef]
29. Furuta, J.; Umebayashi, Y.; Miyamoto, K.; Kikuchi, K.; Otsuka, F.; Sugimura, T.; Ushijima, T. Promoter methylation profiling of 30 genes in human malignant melanoma. *Cancer Sci.* **2004**, *95*, 962–968. [CrossRef]
30. Hoon, D.S.; Spugnardi, M.; Kuo, C.; Huang, S.K.; Morton, D.L.; Taback, B. Profiling epigenetic inactivation of tumor suppressor genes in tumors and plasma from cutaneous melanoma patients. *Oncogene* **2004**, *23*, 4014–4022. [CrossRef]
31. Shen, L.; Kondo, Y.; Guo, Y.; Zhang, J.; Zhang, L.; Ahmed, S.; Shu, J.; Chen, X.; Waterland, R.A.; Issa, J.P. Genome-wide profiling of DNA methylation reveals a class of normally methylated CpG island promoters. *PLoS Genet.* **2007**, *3*, 2023–2036. [CrossRef] [PubMed]
32. Muthusamy, V.; Duraisamy, S.; Bradbury, C.M.; Hobbs, C.; Curley, D.P.; Nelson, B.; Bosenberg, M. Epigenetic silencing of novel tumor suppressors in malignant melanoma. *Cancer Res.* **2006**, *66*, 11187–11193. [CrossRef] [PubMed]
33. Koga, Y.; Pelizzola, M.; Cheng, E.; Krauthammer, M.; Sznol, M.; Ariyan, S.; Narayan, D.; Molinaro, A.M.; Halaban, R.; Weissman, S.M. Genome-wide screen of promoter methylation identifies novel markers in melanoma. *Genome Res.* **2009**, *19*, 1462–1470. [CrossRef] [PubMed]
34. Sigalotti, L.; Covre, A.; Fratta, E.; Parisi, G.; Sonego, P.; Colizzi, F.; Coral, S.; Massarut, S.; Kirkwood, J.M.; Maio, M. Whole genome methylation profiles as independent markers of survival in stage IIIC melanoma patients. *J. Transl. Med.* **2012**, *10*, 185. [CrossRef] [PubMed]
35. Sengupta, D.; Byrum, S.D.; Avaritt, N.L.; Davis, L.; Shields, B.; Mahmoud, F.; Reynolds, M.; Orr, L.M.; Mackintosh, S.G.; Shalin, S.C.; et al. Quantitative Histone Mass Spectrometry Identifies Elevated Histone H3 Lysine 27 (Lys27) Trimethylation in Melanoma. *Mol. Cell. Proteom.* **2016**, *15*, 765–775. [CrossRef] [PubMed]
36. Vire, E.; Brenner, C.; Deplus, R.; Blanchon, L.; Fraga, M.; Didelot, C.; Morey, L.; Van Eynde, A.; Bernard, D.; Vanderwinden, J.M.; et al. The Polycomb group protein EZH2 directly controls DNA methylation. *Nature* **2006**, *439*, 871–874. [CrossRef]
37. Malik, P.; Cashen, A.F. Decitabine in the treatment of acute myeloid leukemia in elderly patients. *Cancer Manag. Res.* **2014**, *6*, 53–61.
38. Young, C.S.; Clarke, K.M.; Kettyle, L.M.; Thompson, A.; Mills, K.I. Decitabine-Vorinostat combination treatment in acute myeloid leukemia activates pathways with potential for novel triple therapy. *Oncotarget* **2017**, *8*, 51429–51446. [CrossRef]
39. Momparler, R.L.; Côté, S.; Momparler, L.F.; Idaghdour, Y. Epigenetic therapy of acute myeloid leukemia using 5-aza-2-deoxycytidine (decitabine) in combination with inhibitors of histone methylation and deacetylation. *Clin. Epigenetics* **2014**, *6*, 19. [CrossRef]
40. Sorm, F.; Vesely, J. Effect of 5-aza-2-deoxycytidine against leukemic and hemopoietic tissues in AKR mice. *Neoplasma* **1968**, *15*, 339–343.
41. Christman, J.K. 5-Azacytidine and 5-aza-2-deoxycytidine as inhibitors of DNA methylation: Mechanistic studies and their implications for cancer therapy. *Oncogene* **2002**, *21*, 5483–5495. [CrossRef] [PubMed]
42. Issa, J.P.; Garcia-Manero, G.; Giles, F.J.; Mannari, R.; Thomas, D.; Faderl, S.; Bayar, E.; Lyons, J.; Rosenfeld, C.S.; Cortes, J.; et al. Phase 1 study of low-dose prolonged exposure schedules of the hypomethylating agent 5-aza-2-deoxycytidine (decitabine) in hematopoietic malignancies. *Blood* **2004**, *103*, 1635–1640. [CrossRef] [PubMed]
43. Rajaii, F.; Asnaghi, L.; Enke, R.; Merbs, S.L.; Handa, J.T.; Eberhart, C.G. The demethylating agent 5-Aza reduces the growth, invasiveness, and clonogenicity of uveal and cutaneous melanoma. *Invest. Ophthalmol. Vis. Sci.* **2014**, *55*, 6178–6186. [CrossRef] [PubMed]
44. El Baroudi, M.; La Sala, D.; Cinti, C.; Capobianco, E. Pathway landscapes and epigenetic regulation in breast cancer and melanoma cell lines. *Theor. Biol. Med. Model.* **2014**, *11*, S8. [CrossRef] [PubMed]
45. Herr, I.; Buchler, M.W. Dietary constituents of broccoli and other cruciferous vegetables: Implications for prevention and therapy of cancer. *Cancer Treat. Rev.* **2010**, *36*, 377–383. [CrossRef]

46. Higdon, J.V.; Delage, B.; Williams, D.E.; Dashwood, R.H. Cruciferous vegetables and human cancer risk: Epidemiologic evidence and mechanistic basis. *Pharm. Res.* **2007**, *55*, 224–236. [CrossRef]
47. Durko, L.; Malecka-Panas, E. Lifestyle Modifications and Colorectal Cancer. *Curr. Colorectal Cancer Rep.* **2014**, *10*, 45–54. [CrossRef]
48. Sestili, P.; Fimognari, C. Cytotoxic and Antitumor Activity of Sulforaphane: The Role of Reactive Oxygen Species. *Biomed. Res. Int.* **2015**, *2015*, 1–9. [CrossRef]
49. Xiao, D.; Powolny, A.A.; Antosiewicz, J.; Hahm, E.R.; Bommareddy, A.; Zeng, Y.; Desai, D.; Amin, S.; Herman-Antosiewicz, A.; Singh, S.V. Cellular responses to cancer chemopreventive agent D,L-sulforaphane in human prostate cancer cells are initiated by mitochondrial reactive oxygen species. *Pharm. Res.* **2009**, *26*, 1729–1738. [CrossRef]
50. Prochaska, H.J.; Santamaria, A.B.; Talalay, P. Rapid detection of inducers of enzymes that protect against carcinogens. *Proc. Natl. Acad. Sci. USA* **1992**, *89*, 2394–2398. [CrossRef]
51. Riedl, M.A.; Saxon, A.; Diaz-Sanchez, D. Oral sulforaphane increases Phase II antioxidant enzymes in the human upper airway. *Clin. Immunol.* **2009**, *130*, 244–251. [CrossRef] [PubMed]
52. Fimognari, C.; Hrelia, P. Sulforaphane as a promising molecule for fighting cancer. *Mutat. Res.* **2007**, *635*, 90–104. [CrossRef] [PubMed]
53. Cho, S.D.; Li, G.; Hu, H.; Jiang, C.; Kang, K.S.; Lee, Y.S.; Kim, S.H.; Lu, J. Involvement of c-Jun N-terminal kinase in G2/M arrest and caspase-mediated apoptosis induced by sulforaphane in DU145 prostate cancer cells. *Nutr. Cancer* **2005**, *52*, 213–224. [CrossRef] [PubMed]
54. Choi, S.; Singh, S.V. Bax and Bak are required for apoptosis induction by sulforaphane, a cruciferous vegetable-derived cancer chemopreventive agent. *Cancer Res.* **2005**, *65*, 2035–2043. [CrossRef] [PubMed]
55. Pledgie-Tracy, A.; Sobolewski, M.D.; Davidson, N.E. Sulforaphane induces cell type-specific apoptosis in human breast cancer cell lines. *Mol. Cancer Ther.* **2007**, *6*, 1013–1021. [CrossRef] [PubMed]
56. Myzak, M.C.; Hardin, K.; Wang, R.; Dashwood, R.H.; Ho, E. Sulforaphane inhibits histone deacetylase activity in BPH-1, LnCaP and PC-3 prostate epithelial cells. *Carcinogenesis* **2006**, *27*, 811–819. [CrossRef]
57. Myzak, M.C.; Tong, P.; Dashwood, W.M.; Dashwood, R.H.; Ho, E. Sulforaphane retards the growth of human PC-3 xenografts and inhibits HDAC activity in human subjects. *Exp. Biol. Med.* **2007**, *232*, 227–234.
58. Wang, X.; Li, Y.; Dai, Y.; Liu, Q.; Ning, S.; Liu, J.; Shen, Z.; Zhu, D.; Jiang, F.; Zhang, J.; et al. Sulforaphane improves chemotherapy efficacy by targeting cancer stem cell-like properties via the miR-124/IL-6R/STAT3 axis. *Sci. Rep.* **2016**, *6*, 36796. [CrossRef]
59. Bose, C.; Awasthi, S.; Sharma, R.; Beneš, H.; Hauer-Jensen, M.; Boerma, M.; Singh, S.P. Sulforaphane potentiates anticancer effects of doxorubicin and attenuates its cardiotoxicity in a breast cancer model. *PLoS ONE* **2018**, *13*, e0193918. [CrossRef]
60. Fan, P.; Zhang, Y.; Liu, L.; Zhao, Z.; Yin, Y.; Xiao, X.; Bauer, N.; Gladkich, J.; Mattern, J.; Gao, C.; et al. Continuous exposure of pancreatic cancer cells to dietary bioactive agents does not induce drug resistance unlike chemotherapy. *Cell Death Dis.* **2016**, *7*, e2246. [CrossRef]
61. Bolger, A.M.; Lohse, M.; Usadel, B. Trimmomatic: A flexible trimmer for Illumina sequence data. *Bioinformatics* **2014**, *30*, 2114–2120. [CrossRef] [PubMed]
62. Trapnell, C.; Pachter, L.; Salzberg, S.L. TopHat: Discovering splice junctions with RNA-Seq. *Bioinformatics* **2009**, *25*, 1105–1111. [CrossRef] [PubMed]
63. Anders, S.; Pyl, P.T.; Huber, W. HTSeq—A Python framework to work with high-throughput sequencing data. *Bioinformatics* **2015**, *31*, 166–169. [CrossRef] [PubMed]
64. Gotz, S.; García-Gómez, J.M.; Terol, J.; Williams, T.D.; Nagaraj, S.H.; Nueda, M.J.; Robles, M.; Talón, M.; Dopazo, J.; Conesa, A. High-throughput functional annotation and data mining with the Blast2GO suite. *Nucleic Acids Res.* **2008**, *36*, 3420–3435. [CrossRef] [PubMed]
65. Robinson, M.D.; Oshlack, A. A scaling normalization method for differential expression analysis of RNA-seq data. *Genome Biol.* **2010**, *11*, R25. [CrossRef] [PubMed]
66. Benjamini, Y.; Hochberg, Y. Controlling The False Discovery Rate-A Practical And Powerful Approach To Multiple Testing. *J. R. Stat. Soc. Ser. B* **1995**, *57*, 289–300. [CrossRef]
67. Taverna, S.D.; Ueberheide, B.M.; Liu, Y.; Tackett, A.J.; Diaz, R.L.; Shabanowitz, J.; Chait, B.T.; Hunt, D.F.; Allis, C.D. Long-distance combinatorial linkage between methylation and acetylation on histone H3 N termini. *Proc. Natl. Acad. Sci. USA* **2007**, *104*, 2086–2091. [CrossRef]

68. El Kennani, S.; Crespo, M.; Govin, J.; Pflieger, D. Proteomic Analysis of Histone Variants and Their PTMs: Strategies and Pitfalls. *Proteomes* **2018**, *6*, 29. [CrossRef]
69. Chiang, T.; Koss, B.; Su, L.; Washam, C.; Byrum, S.; Storey, A.; Tackett, A. Effect of sulforaphane and 5-aza-2′-deoxycytidine on melanoma cell growth. *NCBI: Gene Expression Omnibus*, accession number GSE127252, 2019. Available online: https://www.ncbi.nlm.nih.gov/geo/query/acc.cgi?acc=GSE127252 (accessed on 26 June 2019).
70. Parnaud, G.; Li, P.; Cassar, G.; Rouimi, P.; Tulliez, J.; Combaret, L.; Gamet-Payrastre, L. Mechanism of sulforaphane-induced cell cycle arrest and apoptosis in human colon cancer cells. *Nutr. Cancer* **2004**, *48*, 198–206. [CrossRef]
71. Cheng, Y.M.; Tsai, C.C.; Hsu, Y.C. Sulforaphane, a Dietary Isothiocyanate, Induces G(2)/M Arrest in Cervical Cancer Cells through CyclinB1 Downregulation and GADD45beta/CDC2 Association. *Int. J. Mol. Sci.* **2016**, *17*, 1530. [CrossRef]
72. Alcazar, O.; Achberger, S.; Aldrich, W.; Hu, Z.; Negrotto, S.; Saunthararajah, Y.; Triozzi, P. Epigenetic regulation by decitabine of melanoma differentiation in vitro and in vivo. *Int. J. Cancer* **2012**, *131*, 18–29. [CrossRef] [PubMed]
73. Vijayaraghavalu, S.; Labhasetwar, V. Efficacy of decitabine-loaded nanogels in overcoming cancer drug resistance is mediated via sustained DNA methyltransferase 1 (DNMT1) depletion. *Cancer Lett.* **2013**, *331*, 122–129. [CrossRef] [PubMed]
74. Park, S.L.; Justiniano, R.; Williams, J.D.; Cabello, C.M.; Qiao, S.; Wondrak, G.T. The Tryptophan-Derived Endogenous Aryl Hydrocarbon Receptor Ligand 6-Formylindolo[3,2-b]Carbazole Is a Nanomolar UVA Photosensitizer in Epidermal Keratinocytes. *J. Investig. Derm.* **2015**, *135*, 1649–1658. [CrossRef] [PubMed]
75. Tran, T.T.; Schulman, J.; Fisher, D.E. UV and pigmentation: Molecular mechanisms and social controversies. *Pigment Cell Melanoma Res.* **2008**, *21*, 509–516. [CrossRef] [PubMed]
76. Reichrath, J.; Rass, K. Ultraviolet damage, DNA repair and vitamin D in nonmelanoma skin cancer and in malignant melanoma: An update. *Adv. Exp. Med. Biol.* **2014**, *810*, 208–233. [PubMed]
77. Loetscher, P.; Seitz, M.; Clark-Lewis, I.; Baggiolini, M.; Moser, B. Activation of NK cells by CC chemokines. Chemotaxis, Ca2+ mobilization, and enzyme release. *J. Immunol.* **1996**, *156*, 322–327. [PubMed]
78. Sconocchia, G.; Arriga, R.; Tornillo, L.; Terracciano, L.; Ferrone, S.; Spagnoli, G.C. Melanoma cells inhibit NK cell functions. *Cancer Res.* **2012**, *72*, 5428–5429. [CrossRef]
79. Mgrditchian, T.; Arakelian, T.; Paggetti, J.; Noman, M.Z.; Viry, E.; Moussay, E.; Van Moer, K.; Kreis, S.; Guerin, C.; Buart, S.; et al. Targeting autophagy inhibits melanoma growth by enhancing NK cells infiltration in a CCL5-dependent manner. *Proc. Natl. Acad. Sci. USA* **2017**, *114*, E9271–E9279. [CrossRef]
80. Norris, S.; Coleman, A.; Kuri-Cervantes, L.; Bower, M.; Nelson, M.; Goodier, M.R. PD-1 expression on natural killer cells and CD8(+) T cells during chronic HIV-1 infection. *Viral Immunol.* **2012**, *25*, 329–332. [CrossRef]
81. Stojanovic, A.; Fiegler, N.; Brunner-Weinzierl, M.; Cerwenka, A. CTLA-4 is expressed by activated mouse NK cells and inhibits NK Cell IFN-gamma production in response to mature dendritic cells. *J. Immunol.* **2014**, *192*, 4184–4191. [CrossRef]
82. Noman, M.Z.; Berchem, G.; Janji, B. Targeting autophagy blocks melanoma growth by bringing natural killer cells to the tumor battlefield. *Autophagy* **2018**, *14*, 730–732. [CrossRef] [PubMed]
83. Noman, M.Z.; Paggetti, J.; Moussay, E.; Berchem, G.; Janji, B. Driving Natural Killer cells toward the melanoma tumor battlefield: Autophagy as a valuable therapeutic target. *Oncoimmunology* **2018**, *7*, e1452583. [CrossRef] [PubMed]
84. Bottcher, J.P.; Bonavita, E.; Chakravarty, P.; Blees, H.; Cabeza-Cabrerizo, M.; Sammicheli, S.; Rogers, N.C.; Sahai, E.; Zelenay, S.; Reis e Sousa, C. NK Cells Stimulate Recruitment of cDC1 into the Tumor Microenvironment Promoting Cancer Immune Control. *Cell* **2018**, *172*, 1022–1037. [CrossRef] [PubMed]
85. Benvenuto-Andrade, C.; Oseitutu, A.; Agero, A.L.; Marghoob, A.A. Cutaneous melanoma: Surveillance of patients for recurrence and new primary melanomas. *Derm. Ther.* **2005**, *18*, 423–435. [CrossRef] [PubMed]
86. Faries, M.B.; Steen, S.; Ye, X.; Sim, M.; Morton, D.L. Late recurrence in melanoma: Clinical implications of lost dormancy. *J. Am. Coll. Surg.* **2013**, *217*, 27–34. [CrossRef] [PubMed]

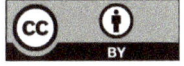

© 2019 by the authors. Licensee MDPI, Basel, Switzerland. This article is an open access article distributed under the terms and conditions of the Creative Commons Attribution (CC BY) license (http://creativecommons.org/licenses/by/4.0/).

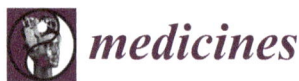

Article

Oral Intake of Royal Jelly Has Protective Effects Against Tyrosine Kinase Inhibitor-Induced Toxicity in Patients with Renal Cell Carcinoma: A Randomized, Double-Blinded, Placebo-Controlled Trial

Kyohei Araki, Yasuyoshi Miyata *, Kojiro Ohba, Yuichiro Nakamura, Tomohiro Matsuo, Yasushi Mochizuki and Hideki Sakai

Department of Urology, Nagasaki University Graduate School of Biomedical Sciences, 1-7-1 Sakamoto, Nagasaki, Nagasaki 852-8501, Japan; k-araki205@cameo.plala.or.jp (K.A.); ohba-k@nagasaki-u.ac.jp (K.O.); yn1238056@yahoo.co.jp (Y.N.); tomozo1228@hotmail.com (T.M.); mochi@nagasaki-u.ac.jp (Y.M.); hsakai@nagasaki-u.ac.jp (H.S.)
* Correspondence: yasu-myt@nagasaki-u.ac.jp; Tel.: +81-95-819-7340

Received: 5 December 2018; Accepted: 18 December 2018; Published: 20 December 2018

Abstract: Background: Although tyrosine kinase inhibitors (TKIs) are still recommended as the standard therapy in renal cell carcinoma (RCC), the high frequency of adverse events is a weakness of this therapy. Because royal jelly (RJ) possesses anti-inflammatory and antioxidant properties, we assessed its protective effects on TKI-induced toxicities in RCC patients. **Methods:** We enrolled 33 patients with advanced RCC who were assigned to start TKI therapy in combination with a randomized, double-blinded, placebo-controlled RJ trial consisting of a placebo group with 17 subjects and an RJ group with 16 subjects. **Results:** Fatigue and anorexia frequencies in the RJ group were significantly lower than in the placebo group (p = 0.003 and 0.015, respectively). A statistically significant correlation between RJ and fatigue or anorexia was detected in sunitinib-treated patients. The dose reduction- or discontinuation-free periods were significantly longer (p = 0.013) in the RJ group than in the placebo group. Furthermore, similar observations were made in sunitinib-treated patients (p = 0.016). **Conclusions:** Our clinical trial showed that RJ exerted protective effects against TKI-induced fatigue and anorexia and lowered TKI dose reduction or discontinuation. Hence, RJ is beneficial for maintaining the quality of life and medication compliance in TKI-treated RCC patients.

Keywords: royal jelly; adverse events; tyrosine kinase inhibitors; renal cell carcinoma; double-blinded; randomized clinical trial

1. Introduction

Renal cell carcinoma (RCC) is one of the most common urological cancers, and its incidence has continuously increased over the past few decades [1]. Although a nephrectomy is usually performed for organ-confined RCC, additional systematic therapy is the standard treatment strategy in patients with metastatic RCC. Currently, new treatment options including immune check-point inhibitors are being developed; however, a molecularly targeted therapy using tyrosine kinase inhibitors (TKIs) is still the recommended standard therapy for these patients [2–4]. In addition, molecularly targeted therapies are often used as neoadjuvant therapy for cytoreductive nephrectomy [5], and clinical trials of combination therapies including molecularly targeted therapeutics and other anticancer agents are currently in progress [6–8]. On the other hand, a major limitation of molecularly targeted therapies is the relatively high frequency of adverse events (AEs) with occasionally severe effects [9,10]. Therefore, the management of drug-induced AEs is critical for maintaining the quality of life during treatment and continuous therapy in these patients.

Sunitinib and pazopanib are approved as first-line therapy for patients with RCC, especially in favorable- or intermediate-risk clear cell RCC [2]. In addition, these TKIs are often used in real-world patients with non-clear cell RCC [11]. On the other hand, axitinib and sorafenib are also used in some patients with metastatic RCC [12,13]. Typical AEs linked to these TKIs include various symptoms such as oral mucositis, hand–foot syndrome, hypertension, fatigue, and gastrointestinal events [14–18]. In addition, functional disorders of the kidneys, liver, and thyroid are often associated with TKIs [14,15,17]. The occurrence and progression of these AEs are suggested to be mediated by complex mechanisms that involve inflammation, oxidative stress, and the immune system [19–21]. Based on these findings, we hypothesized that controlling these biological factors may suppress TKI-induced adverse events.

Royal jelly (RJ) is secreted by the hypopharyngeal and mandibular glands of worker honeybees of *Apis mellifera*, and is the exclusive food for the queen honeybee and larvae. The most important biological effects of RJ are its anti-inflammatory and antioxidative activities, and its ability to exert some control over the immune system [22–24]. These RJ-related activities are predicted to be beneficial in the protection against anticancer agent-induced adverse events involving inflammation, oxidative stress, and immune system dysfunction [25,26]. In fact, the protective efficacy of RJ against anticancer therapy associated toxic effects, such as oral mucositis, intestinal damage, and nephro- and hepato-toxicities, has been demonstrated in animal models with malignancies [27–30].

Thus, in recent decades, several studies have examined the biological effects of RJ on cancer cell lines and corresponding animal models. However, despite several clinical trials, not many studies have reported the clinical benefits and limitations of RJ administration in cancer patients [31–35]. Specifically, there are no reports about the effects of RJ on the adverse events caused by molecularly targeted therapies in RCC patients. Therefore, the aim of this study was to assess the protective efficacy of RJ against TKI-induced toxicities in patients with RCC.

2. Methods

2.1. Patients

This study protocol was approved by the Human Ethics Review Committee of Nagasaki University Hospital (Nagasaki, Japan; No. 15102604-2), and it was registered as UMIN000020152. In addition, this trial was conducted according to the Declaration of Helsinki. Patients provided written informed consent to participate in all aspects of the study. Patients with RCC who had been assigned to start TKIs were enrolled by the Nagasaki University Hospital. Eligibility criteria of this trial were age >20 years, Eastern Cooperative Oncology Group performance status (ECOG PS) 0 or 1, and no honey allergy.

2.2. Study Design

This is a randomized, double-blinded, placebo-controlled clinical trial. Patients were assigned to two groups, namely the placebo and RJ groups, at a ratio of 1:1 using computer-generated random numbers. The patient selection process was performed by independent non-medical staff at our hospital who had no information on the aim of this trial, and the process was also hidden from the patients and urologists who provided treatment until the end of all analyses.

RJ and the placebo were provided by the Yamada Agriculture Center Inc (Okayama, Japan). RJ and the placebo were prepared as capsules containing 900 mg RJ and starch, respectively, that share the same taste, smell, size, shape, and color. Capsules were orally administered four times per day for three months.

2.3. Protocol

All subjects received medical examinations and were checked for clinical symptoms every two weeks. Blood samples were collected simultaneously every two weeks and subjected to laboratory analysis routinely performed in patients treated with TKIs. The initial starting dose of sunitinib, pazopanib, axitinib, and sunitinib was 50 mg/day, 800 mg/day, 10 mg/day, and 800 mg/day, respectively, but if an intolerable AE was observed, the dose was decreased to 37.5 mg/day, 400–600 mg/day, 5 mg/day, and 400 mg/day, respectively. In addition, for the sunitinib regimen, if the dose reduction was necessary, all affected patients were treated with an alternative every other day [36]. Furthermore, TKI administration was stopped if intolerable AEs persisted or high-grade abnormalities in the blood analysis were observed. The primary outcome was the frequency and severity of AEs caused by TKIs in patients with RCC, and the secondary outcome was the sustained period of the initial TKI regimen.

Toxicities were graded according to the National Cancer Institute Common Terminology Criteria for Adverse Events, version 5.0. In this study, toxicities classified as grade 3 and 4, or identified as the cause for discontinued TKI administration, were judged as severe AEs.

2.4. Statistical Analyses

Results are expressed as the mean and standard deviation (SD) for normally distributed data and the median and interquartile range (IQR) for non-normally distributed data. The Student's t-test or Mann–Whitney U test was used to compare continuous variables and Scheffé's method was used for multiple comparisons. The sustained periods of initial dosage were derived from Kaplan–Meier curves, and statistical significance was analyzed using the log-rank test. Values with $p < 0.05$ were considered statistically significant. Statistical analyses were carried out using StatView for Windows v.5.0 software (Abacus Concept, Berkeley, CA, USA).

3. Results

All subjects of the placebo and RJ group consumed the respective capsules for three months or until disease progression. In addition, we confirmed that the compliance rate was >95% in both groups and no patient experienced any side effects including allergy due to the trial capsules.

3.1. Patient Background

Thirty-three patients with RCC were enrolled in this study. The pathological features and basic characteristics of our study population at baseline are presented in Table 1.

Table 1. Clinicopathological features and basic characteristics.

Variables	Entire (n = 33)	Placebo (n = 17)	Royal Jelly (n = 16)	p Value
Age				0.101
Mean ± SD, years	67.6 ± 6.6	65.8 ± 8.8	69.6 ± 5.9	
Gender; n (%)				0.909
Male/Female	23/10 (30.3)	12/5 (29.4)	11/5 (31.3)	
Performance Status				0.598
0/1	16/17 (51.5)	9/8 (47.1)	7/9 (56.3)	
Pathological Type				0.446
Conventional	29 (87.9)	16 (94.1)	13 (81.3)	
Fuhrman Grade				0.425
1 or 2/3 or 4	6/27 (81.8)	2/15 (88.2)	4/12 (75.0)	
pT stage				0.201
1 or 2/3 or 4	9/24 (72.7)	3/14 (82.4)	6/10 (62.5)	
Lymph Node Metastasis				0.881
Presence	19 (57.6)	10 (58.8)	9 (56.3)	
Distant Metastasis				0.325
Presence	27 (81.8)	15 (88.2)	12 (75.0)	
Neo-Adjuvant Setting				0.965
Yes	2 (6.1)	1 (5.9)	1 (6.3)	

Table 1. Cont.

Variables	Entire (n = 33)	Placebo (n = 17)	Royal Jelly (n = 16)	p Value
Past Therapy Used TKI				0.948
Presence	4 (12.1)	2 (11.8)	2 (12.5)	
TKIs				0.539
Sunitinib	21 (63.6)	11 (64.7)	10 (62.5)	
Pazopanib	7 (21.2)	3 (17.6)	4 (25.0)	
Axitinib	4 (12.1)	3 (17.6)	1 (6.3)	
Sorafenib	1 (3.0)	0 (0.0)	1 (6.3)	

TKIs = tyrosine kinase inhibitors. SD = standard deviation.

The statistical analysis indicated that the baseline parameters did not significantly differ between the placebo and the RJ groups. As shown in Table 1, among the 33 patients, 21, 8, and 3 patients were treated with sunitinib, pazopanib, and axitinib, respectively, whereas only one patient was treated with sorafenib. The patients were further divided into two subgroups, namely the sunitinib and the other TKI group, because 63.5% of the patients were treated with sunitinib. The clinicopathological features and basic characteristics of each subgroup are listed in Table 2.

Table 2. Clinicopathological features and basic characteristics according to used agents.

Variables	Placebo	Royal Jelly	p Value
Sunitinib	n = 11	n = 10	
Age (mean ± SD), years	66.5 ± 8.3	67.8 ± 5.8	0.673
Gender; Male/Female, n (%)	6/5 (45.5)	8/2 (20.0)	0.217
Performance Status; 0/1	7/4 (36.4)	6/4 (40.0)	0.864
Pathological Type; Conventional	11 (100.0)	8 (80.0)	0.297
Fuhrman grade; 2/3+4	1/10 (90.9)	2/8 (80.0)	0.476
pT stage; 1+2/3+4	2/9 (81.8)	3/7 (70.0)	0.525
Lymph Node Metastasis; Presence	7 (63.6)	6 (60.0)	0.864
Distant Metastasis; Presence	9 (81.8)	8 (80.0)	0.916
Neo-Adjuvant Setting; Yes	1 (9.1)	0 (0.0)	0.329
Past Therapy Used TKI; Presence	1 (9.1)	0 (0.0)	0.329
Others	n = 6	n = 6	
Age (mean ± SD); years	64.5 ± 3.8	72.5 ± 5.3	0.013
Gender; Male / Female	6/0 (0.0)	3/3 (50.0)	0.182
Performance Status; 0/1	2/4 (66.7)	1/5 (83.3)	0.505
Pathological Type; Conventional	5 (83.3)	5 (83.3)	0.999
Fuhrman grade; 2/3+4	1/5 (83.3)	3/3 (50.0)	0.221
pT Stage; 1+2/3+4	1/5 (83.3)	2/4 (66.7)	0.501
LN Metastasis; Presence	3 (50.0)	3 (50.0)	0.999
Distant Metastasis; Presence	6 (100.0)	4 (66.7)	0.121
Neo-Adjuvant Setting; Yes	0 (0.0)	1 (16.7)	0.296
Past Therapy Used TKI; Presence	1 (16.7)	2 (33.3)	0.505

In the other TKI group, the mean age of the RJ group was significantly higher ($p = 0.013$) compared to that of the RJ group. However, the remaining parameters did not significantly vary between these two groups.

3.2. Adverse Events

In the study population ($n = 33$), the most common AE was hypertension ($n = 23$; 69.7%) followed by fatigue ($n = 20$; 60.6%), and anorexia ($n = 18$; 60.0%) and hand–foot syndrome ($n = 18$; 60.0%). Furthermore, anorexia ($n = 4$; 12.1%) was the most common severe adverse event.

As shown in Table 3, the frequencies and severities of fatigue and anorexia were significantly lower in the RJ group than those in the placebo group ($p = 0.003$ and 0.015, respectively). The digestive symptoms varied similarly, but the difference between the RJ and placebo group was not statistically significant ($p = 0.077$). In addition, none of the other symptoms varied significantly, including hypertension. However, when the same analysis was performed separately on the subgroups of patients treated with either sunitinib or other TKIs, such significant differences in fatigue and anorexia differed significantly between the RJ and placebo groups in patients treated with sunitinib ($p = 0.040$ and 0.038, respectively), but not in those treated with other TKIs ($p = 0.065$ and 0.343, respectively). The frequencies of the remaining symptoms were similar between the two groups regardless of the TKI regimen.

Table 3. Relationships between royal jelly intake and clinical symptoms.

Adverse Events	Entire		Sunitinib		Others	
	Placebo (n = 17)	RJ (n = 16)	Placebo (n = 11)	RJ (n = 10)	Placebo (n = 6)	RJ (n = 6)
Hypertension						
Nothing	6 (35.3)	4 (25.0)	5 (45.5)	3 (30.0)	1 (16.7)	1 (16.7)
Mild	10 (58.8)	12 (75.0)	6 (54.5)	7 (70.0)	4 (66.7)	5 (83.3)
Severe	1 (5.9)	0 (0.0)	0 (0.0)	0 (0.0)	1 (16.7)	0 (0.0)
p value	0.460		0.466		0.574	
Fatigue						
Nothing	2 (11.8)	11 (68.8)	1 (9.1)	6 (60.0)	1 (16.7)	5 (83.3)
Mild	13 (76.5)	5 (31.3)	9 (81.8)	4 (40.0)	4 (66.7)	1 (16.7)
Severe	2 (11.8)	0 (0.0)	1 (9.1)	0 (0.0)	1 (16.7)	0 (0.0)
p value	0.003		0.040		0.065	
Anorexia						
Nothing	4 (23.5)	11 (68.8)	3 (27.3)	8 (80.0)	1 (16.7)	3 (50.0)
Mild	9 (52.9)	5 (31.3)	5 (45.5)	2 (20.0)	4 (66.7)	3 (50.0)
Severe	4 (23.5)	0 (0.0)	3 (27.3)	0 (0.0)	1 (16.7)	0 (0.0)
p value	0.015		0.038		0.343	
Digestive Symptoms						
Nothing	6 (35.3)	11 (68.8)	3 (27.3)	7 (70.0)	3 (50.0)	4 (66.7)
Mild	8 (47.1)	5 (31.3)	6 (54.5)	3 (30.0)	2 (33.3)	2 (33.3)
Severe	3 (17.6)	0 (0.0)	2 (18.2)	0 (0.0)	1 (16.7)	0 (0.0)
p value	0.077		0.102		0.565	
Dysgeusia						
Nothing	7 (41.2)	9 (56.3)	5 (45.5)	5 (50.0)	2 (33.3)	4 (66.7)
Mild	9 (52.9)	7 (43.8)	5 (45.5)	5 (50.0)	4 (66.7)	2 (33.3)
Severe	1 (5.9)	0 (0.0)	1 (9.1)	0 (0.0)	0 (0.0)	0 (0.0)
p value	0.479		0.621		0.248	
Hand–Foot Syndrome						
Nothing	7 (41.2)	8 (50.0)	3 (27.3)	4 (40.0)	4 (66.7)	4 (66.7)
Mild	9 (52.9)	8 (50.0)	8 (72.7))	6 (60.0)	1 (16.7)	2 (33.3)
Severe	1 (5.9)	0 (0.0)	0 (0.0)	0 (0.0)	1 (16.7)	0 (0.0)
p value	0.578		0.537		0.513	
Oral Mucositis						
Nothing	9 (52.9)	11 (68.8)	7 (63.6)	7 (70.0)	2 (33.3)	4 (66.7)
Mild	8 (47.1)	5 (31.3)	4 (36.4)	3 (30.0)	4 (66.7)	2 (33.3)
Severe	0 (0.0)	0 (0.0)	0 (0.0)	0 (0.0)	0 (0.0)	0 (0.0)
p value	0.353		0.757		0.248	

RJ = royal jelly.

Table 4 shows the laboratory blood test results in relation to the trial capsule treatment groups. The frequency of patients with normal anemia values was higher in the RJ group (87.5%) than in the placebo group (58.8%); however, the difference was not statistically significant ($p = 0.162$). When the same analysis was performed with the data of the sunitinib-treated patients, no significant difference was detected ($p = 0.117$). Overall, none of the laboratory blood test results varied significantly between the placebo and the RJ group (Table 4).

Table 4. Relationships between royal jelly intake and results of blood examinations.

Adverse Events	Entire		Sunitinib		Others	
	Placebo (n = 17)	RJ (n = 16)	Placebo (n = 11)	RJ (n = 10)	Placebo (n = 6)	RJ (n = 6)
Leukopenia						
Nothing	11 (35.3)	11 (25.0)	5 (45.5)	6 (60.0)	6 (100.0)	5 (83.3)
Low	5 (58.8)	5 (75.0)	5 (45.5)	4 (40.0)	0 (0.0)	1 (16.7)
High	1 (5.9)	0 (0.0)	1 (9.1)	0 (0.0)	0 (0.0)	0 (0.0)
p value	0.616		0.561		0.296	
Anemia						
Nothing	10 (58.8)	14 (87.5)	4 (36.4)	8 (80.0)	6 (100.0)	6 (100.0)
Mild	6 (35.3)	2 (12.5)	4 (36.4)	2 (20.0)	0 (0.0)	0 (0.0)
Severe	1 (5.9)	0 (0.0)	1 (9.1)	0 (0.0)	0 (0.0)	0 (0.0)
p value	0.162		0.117		>0.999	
Platelets						
Nothing	5 (29.4)	9 (56.3)	2 (18.2)	5 (50.0)	3 (50.0)	4 (66.7)
Mild	8 (47.1)	4 (25.0)	6 (54.5)	3 (30.0)	2 (33.3)	1 (16.7)
Severe	4 (23.5)	3 (18.8)	3 (27.3)	2 (20.0)	1 (16.7)	1 (16.7)
p value	0.274		0.295		0.788	
Renal Dysfunction						
Nothing	8 (47.1)	10 (62.5)	5 (45.5)	6 (60.0)	3 (50.0)	4 (66.7)
Mild	9 (52.9)	6 (37.5)	6 (54.5)	4 (40.0)	3 (50.0)	2 (33.3)
Severe	0 (0.0)	0 (0.0)	0 (0.0)	0 (0.0)	0 (0.0)	0 (0.0)
p value	0.373		0.505		0.558	
Liver Dysfunction						
Nothing	12 (70.6)	14 (87.5)	7 (63.6)	9 (90.0)	5 (83.3)	5 (83.3)
Mild	4 (23.5)	1 (6.3)	4 (36.4)	1 (10.0)	0 (0.0)	0 (0.0)
Severe	1 (5.9)	1 (6.3)	0 (0.0)	0 (0.0)	1 (16.7)	1 (16.7)
p value	0.382		0.621		0.999	
Thyroid Abnormality						
Nothing	9 (52.9)	10 (62.5)	7 (63.6)	7 (70.0)	2 (33.3)	3 (50.0)
Mild	7 (41.2)	6 (37.5)	4 (36.4)	3 (30.0)	3 (50.0)	3 (50.0)
Severe	1 (5.9)	0 (0.0)	0 (0.0)	0 (0.0)	1 (16.7)	0 (0.0)
P value	0.577		0.757		0.549	

3.3. Dose Reduction or Discontinuation of Tyrosine Kinase Inhibitors

In our study population, 23 of the 33 patients (69.7%) required a dose reduction or discontinuation of the TKI regimen due to severe AEs and disease progression within three months of TKI treatment initiation. The frequency of dose reduction or discontinuation was significantly lower ($p = 0.017$) in the RJ group (5/16 = 50.0%) than in the placebo group (15/17 = 88.2%). The Kaplan–Meier survival curves for dose-reduction- or discontinuation-free survival rates in the placebo and RJ group are shown in Figure 1A. The free-periods were significantly longer ($p = 0.013$) in the RJ group than in the placebo group. Furthermore, a similar result was observed in patients treated with sunitinib ($p = 0.016$; Figure 1B). However, although the dose-reduction- or discontinuation-free survival rates appeared to be better in the RJ group than in the placebo group among patients treated with TKIs other than sunitinib, the difference between these subgroups was not significant ($p = 0.296$; Figure 1C).

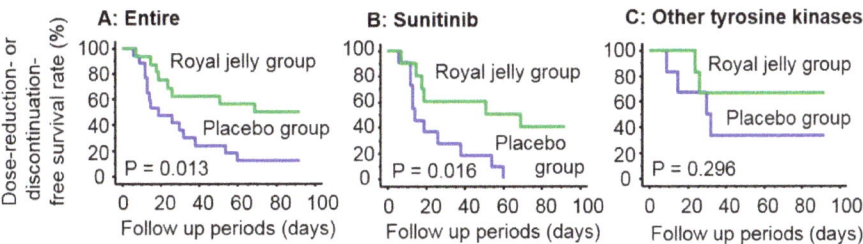

Figure 1. Kaplan–Meier survival curves of the dose-reduction- or discontinuation-free survival rate in the placebo and RJ groups. Dose-reduction- or discontinuation-free survival was better in the RJ group than in the placebo group for patients treated with any TKI (**A**) and sunitinib (**B**) ($p = 0.127$ and 0.016, respectively). However, this difference was not observed in patients treated with other TKIs (**C**).

4. Discussion

In this study, we investigated the preventive effects of prophylactic RJ consumption on AEs associated with TKI-induced toxicities because the appropriate management of these AEs is critical for maintaining quality of life in RCC patients treated with TKIs. Various harmful symptoms and abnormal observations are known as adverse events of TKIs [12,14–18]. Among these chemotherapy-induced symptoms, such as oral mucositis, anorexia, digestive symptoms, fatigue, and damage of the kidneys and liver, few have been shown to be suppressed by RJ administration in animal experiments and clinical trials [27–34,37]. In addition, it is known that RJ improves protection against hypertension, hand–foot syndrome, and bone marrow suppression, which are representative adverse events associated with TKIs [38,39]. However, we found that among these harmful symptoms, RJ administration was not significantly associated with the frequency and severity of hypertension, hand–foot syndrome, oral mucositis, dysgeusia, and kidney or liver damage. Importantly, we demonstrated that fatigue and anorexia in the RJ group were significantly mild compared to that in the placebo group. Interestingly, RJ has been shown to exert anti-fatigue effects in an animal experiment that investigated fatigue-related parameters such as serum lactate, serum ammonia, and muscle glycogen after swimming in mice treated with RJ [40]. The study found that these parameters were improved by RJ intake [40]. However, we should note that this fatigue was not induced by anticancer therapies such as TKIs. However, there is a report that processed honey and RJ ameliorated cancer-related fatigue in a double-blinded, randomized clinical trial [33]. Specifically, the visual analogue fatigue scale and fatigue severity score in the test article group (processed honey and RJ for four weeks; $n = 26$) were significantly lower than those in the control group (pure honey for four weeks; $n = 26$) [33]. We believe that the present study supports this previous result. However, the previous study had some limitations; for example, the study population included six different types of cancer (breast, gastric, esophageal, colon, rectal, and prostate cancer). Although there was no statistical difference between the composition of the study and control group, the patients had to be treated with four different methods (hormonal therapy, chemotherapy, chemoradiation, and radiotherapy). Furthermore, as discussed by the authors, the short duration of intervention (four weeks) was another limitation [33]. Thus, the present study is the first report on the association between RJ and cancer-related fatigue in RCC patients treated with TKIs. Fatigue is widely recognized as a highly common adverse event in TKI-treated patients with metastatic RCC (sunitinib, 55%; pazopanib, 27%; axitinib, 9%; and sorafenib; 8%) [12]. In addition, it was observed that only 4% of these patients received pharmacologic treatment for fatigue, whereas 72% of hypertension was treated [12]. Moreover, there are only a few effective treatment options for fatigue caused by TKIs. Hence, our observation that RJ may significantly suppress TKI-induced fatigue is an important finding for TKI-based treatment strategies.

In addition to fatigue, our results demonstrated that RJ suppressed the frequency and severity of anorexia. To our knowledge, this is the first report about the preventive effect of RJ on anorexia in RCC patients. In addition, there is no information on the relationship between RJ and anorexia in patients with malignancies. In general, anorexia in cancer patients is caused by complex interactions involving various factors, such as nausea, constipation, pain, depression, and hypothyroidism [41]. In addition, it is recommended that anorexia treatment should include drugs that target the following conditions: nutritional disorders, muscle catabolism, anemia, and fatigue [42]. Furthermore, it was reported that inflammatory status, oxidative stress, and immunosuppression are important targets for anorexia treatment. From our results, we cannot describe the interactions induced by RJ to exert the preventive effects against anorexia. However, we speculate that there are multiple beneficial effects of RJ on various TKI-induced adverse events including fatigue, digestive symptoms, anemia, and nephro- and hepato-toxicities that contribute to this finding, although RJ is not significantly associated with the prevention of these events. Furthermore, RJ has been reported to possess anti-inflammatory and antioxidative activities, and act as a significant regulator of immune conditions caused by anticancer therapies [35]. We agree with the opinion that the clinical management of anorexia requires a multidisciplinary and multi-pharmacological approach [42]. As useful information for TKI-treatment management, RJ intake is beneficial to prevent anorexia in cancer patients treated with sunitinib.

Our results showed that RJ had no significant effect on oral mucositis. However, a preliminary study designed as a randomized, single-blinded (physician-blinded) trial showed that prophylactic RJ use led to a significant reduction in head and neck cancer patients. However, the study population was small (the RJ and control groups had seven and six patients, respectively) [32]. On the other hand, other investigators also reported that RJ improved symptoms of oral mucositis and shortened the healing time in 103 patients [31]. However, in these two studies, patients were treated with a combination of chemotherapy and radiotherapy. We believe that RJ may prevent the oral mucositis caused by chemotherapy and/or radiotherapy, but not by TKIs.

Our results showed that there was no significant relationship between RJ consumption and the blood test results. Several in vivo studies demonstrated RJ administration led to the protection of various organ functions [35]. For example, RJ strongly suppressed clinical and pathological aggravation of the liver, kidneys, and testis in experimental animals treated with cisplatin [29,30,37]. On the other hand, in a human trial, the serum levels of creatinine and urea were significantly increased during the first and second cycle of cisplatin-based chemotherapy in 32 cancer patients, but the increase in kidney function-related parameters was suppressed by RJ administration. However, the nephroprotective activity was not statistically significant [34]. Our results are similar to those reported in this study, and we assume that differences such as species, dosage, and period of RJ treatment as well as physiological characteristics of the kidneys are causes for the different observations in animal models and cancer patients.

Our study design has several limitations that restrict the conclusions about the preventive effects of RJ on AEs caused by TKIs in patients with RCC. First, the trial had a relatively small number of patients in each group. However, we emphasize that this trial is a preliminary study on the RJ consumption by patients with malignancy treated with TKIs. In addition, the number of patients in the present study appears to be relatively similar to that reported in previous clinical trials on RJ administration [32,33]. Second, the RJ capsules were provided by a company that sells supplements made from honey. To ensure that the study is not biased, we performed this trial as a double-blinded, randomized study, and the administration, data collection, and analysis were done by a third party approved by the Human Ethics Review Committee. Therefore, our results were not affected by the company and we did not receive any financial support for the publication of this manuscript. Finally, our study design cannot identify the active substance causing the beneficial functions of RJ. Although RJ contains mostly sugars, lipids, amino acids, and vitamins, 10-hydroxy-2-decenoic acid (10-HDA), royalisin, and apisin are known as major components with pharmacological activities [43–45]. We assume that some of these RJ-specific components may cause the observed effects. Further detailed analyses are necessary to identify the active ingredients.

In conclusion, our results demonstrated that prophylactic RJ intake is effective for the prevention and suppression of sunitinib-induced fatigue and anorexia. In addition, RJ did not affect treatment safety and compliance. Specifically, we found that the risk of TKI dose reduction or discontinuation was significantly lower in the RJ group than in the placebo group. Sunitinib remains a recommended standard agent used singly or in combination with immune therapy, low molecular weight heparin, and vaccines for the treatment of metastatic RCC [6,7]. Therefore, we believe that our results are important to improve the treatment strategies for RCC. On the other hand, we emphasize that further detailed clinical studies with more participants are needed to determine whether RJ intake prevents TKI-induced AEs in cancer patients.

Author Contributions: Conceptualization: Y.M.; Data Curation: K.O., Y.M.; Formal Analysis: T.M.; Funding acquisition: Y.M.; Investigation: Y.M., K.A., Y.N.; Methodology: K.A., K.O., Y.N.; Supervision: H.S.; Writing—original draft Preparation: K.A., Y.M.; Writing—review and editing: H.S.; All authors agree with the final version of the manuscript. The authors declare that the content of this paper has not been published or submitted for publication elsewhere.

Funding: This study was supported in part by a YAMADA RESEARCH GRANT (to Y.M.).

Acknowledgments: The authors thank Dr. Yuji Sagara for providing technical support.

Conflicts of Interest: The authors declare no conflict of interest.

References

1. Siegel, R.L.; Miller, K.D.; Jemal, A. Cancer statistics, 2017. *CA Cancer J. Clin.* **2017**, *67*, 7–30. [CrossRef] [PubMed]
2. Bedke, J.; Gauler, T.; Grünwald, V.; Hegele, A.; Herrmann, E.; Hinz, S.; Janssen, J.; Schmitz, S.; Schostak, M.; Tesch, H.; et al. Systemic therapy in metastatic renal cell carcinoma. *World J. Urol.* **2017**, *35*, 179–188. [CrossRef] [PubMed]
3. Lai, Y.; Zhao, Z.; Zeng, T.; Liang, X.; Chen, D.; Duan, X.; Zeng, G.; Wu, W. Crosstalk between VEGFR and other receptor tyrosine kinases for TKI therapy of metastatic renal cell carcinoma. *Cancer Cell Int.* **2018**, *18*, 31. [CrossRef] [PubMed]
4. Zarrabi, K.; Wu, S. Current and emerging therapeutic targets for metastatic renal cell carcinoma. *Curr. Oncol. Rep.* **2018**, *20*, 41. [CrossRef] [PubMed]
5. Pooleri, G.K.; Nair, T.B.; Sanjeevan, K.V.; Thomas, A. Neo adjuvant treatment with targeted molecules for renal cell cancer in current clinical practise. *Indian J. Surg. Oncol.* **2012**, *3*, 114–119. [CrossRef]
6. Rizzo, M.; Porta, C. Sunitinib in the treatment of renal cell carcinoma: An update on recent evidence. *Ther. Adv. Urol.* **2017**, *9*, 195–207. [CrossRef]
7. Wentink, M.Q.; Verheul, H.M.W.; Pal, S.K.; George, S.; Voortman, J.; Danchaivijitr, P.; Adelaiye, R.; Poslinski, D.; Groman, A.; Hutson, A.; et al. Phase I Study of dalteparin in combination with sunitinib in patients with metastatic clear cell renal carcinoma. *Clin. Genitourin Cancer* **2017**. [CrossRef]
8. Atkins, M.B.; Plimack, E.R.; Puzanov, I.; Fishman, M.N.; McDermott, D.F.; Cho, D.C.; Vaishampayan, U.; George, S.; Olencki, T.E.; Tarazi, J.C.; et al. Axitinib in combination with pembrolizumab in patients with advanced renal cell cancer: A non-randomised, open-label, dose-finding, and dose-expansion phase 1b trial. *Lancet Oncol.* **2018**, *19*, 405–415. [CrossRef]
9. Clarke, J.M.; George, D.J.; Lisi, S.; Salama, A. Immune checkpoint blockade: The new frontier in cancer treatment. *Target Oncol.* **2018**, *13*, 1–20. [CrossRef]
10. Guo, J.; Jin, J.; Oya, M.; Uemura, H.; Takahashi, S.; Tatsugami, K.; Rha, S.Y.; Lee, J.L.; Chung, J.; Lim, H.Y.; et al. Safety of pazopanib and sunitinib in treatment-naive patients with metastatic renal cell carcinoma: Asian versus non-Asian subgroup analysis of the COMPARZ trial. *J. Hematol. Oncol.* **2018**, *11*, 69. [CrossRef] [PubMed]
11. Fernández-Pello, S.; Hofmann, F.; Tahbaz, R.; Marconi, L.; Lam, T.B.; Albiges, L.; Bensalah, K.; Canfield, S.E.; Dabestani, S.; Giles, R.H.; et al. A systematic review and meta-analysis comparing the effectiveness and adverse effects of different systemic treatments for non-clear cell renal cell carcinoma. *Eur. Urol.* **2017**, *71*, 426–436. [CrossRef] [PubMed]
12. Srinivas, S.; Stein, D.; Teltsch, D.Y.; Tao, S.; Cisar, L.; Ramaswamy, K. Real-world chart review study of adverse events management in patients taking tyrosine kinase inhibitors to treat metastatic renal cell carcinoma. *J. Oncol. Pharm. Pract.* **2018**, *24*, 574–583. [CrossRef] [PubMed]
13. Sheng, X.; Bi, F.; Ren, X.; Cheng, Y.; Wang, J.; Rosbrook, B.; Jiang, M.; Guo, J. First-line axitinib versus sorafenib in Asian patients with metastatic renal cell carcinoma: Exploratory subgroup analyses of Phase III data. *Future Oncol.* **2018**, in press. [CrossRef] [PubMed]
14. Méndez-Vidal, M.J.; Martínez Ortega, E.; Montesa Pino, A.; Pérez Valderrama, B.; Viciana, R. Management of adverse events of targeted therapies in normal and special patients with metastatic renal cell carcinoma. *Cancer Metastasis Rev.* **2012**, *31*, S19–27. [CrossRef] [PubMed]

15. Escudier, B.; Porta, C.; Bono, P.; Powles, T.; Eisen, T.; Sternberg, C.N.; Gschwend, J.E.; De Giorgi, U.; Parikh, O.; Hawkins, R.; et al. Randomized, controlled, double-blind, cross-over trial assessing treatment preference for pazopanib versus sunitinib in patients with metastatic renal cell carcinoma: PISCES Study. *J. Clin. Oncol.* **2014**, *32*, 1412–1418. [CrossRef] [PubMed]
16. Santoni, M.; Conti, A.; De Giorgi, U.; Iacovelli, R.; Pantano, F.; Burattini, L.; Muzzonigro, G.; Berardi, R.; Santini, D.; Cascinu, S. Risk of gastrointestinal events with sorafenib, sunitinib and pazopanib in patients with solid tumors: A systematic review and meta-analysis of clinical trials. *Int. J. Cancer* **2014**, *135*, 763–773. [CrossRef]
17. Chrisoulidou, A.; Mandanas, S.; Margaritidou, E.; Mathiopoulou, L.; Boudina, M.; Georgopoulos, K.; Pazaitou-Panayiotou, K. Treatment compliance and severe adverse events limit the use of tyrosine kinase inhibitors in refractory thyroid cancer. *Onco. Targets Ther.* **2015**, *8*, 2435–2442.
18. Que, Y.; Liang, Y.; Zhao, J.; Ding, Y.; Peng, R.; Guan, Y.; Zhang, X. Treatment-related adverse effects with pazopanib, sorafenib and sunitinib in patients with advanced soft tissue sarcoma: A pooled analysis. *Cancer Manag. Res.* **2018**, *10*, 2141–2150. [CrossRef] [PubMed]
19. Santoni, M.; Rizzo, M.; Burattini, L.; Farfariello, V.; Berardi, R.; Santoni, G.; Carteni, G.; Cascinu, S. Present and future of tyrosine kinase inhibitors in renal cell carcinoma: Analysis of hematologic toxicity. *Recent Pat. Antiinfect. Drug Discov.* **2012**, *7*, 104–110. [CrossRef] [PubMed]
20. Gopal, S.; Miller, K.B.; Jaffe, I.Z. Molecular mechanisms for vascular complications of targeted cancer therapies. *Clin. Sci. (Lond.)* **2016**, *130*, 1763–1779. [CrossRef] [PubMed]
21. Teppo, H.R.; Soini, Y.; Karihtala, P. Reactive oxygen species-mediated mechanisms of action of targeted cancer therapy. *Oxid. Med. Cell. Longev.* **2017**, *2017*, 1485283. [CrossRef] [PubMed]
22. Liu, J.R.; Yang, Y.C.; Shi, L.S.; Peng, C.C. Antioxidant properties of royal jelly associated with larval age and time of harvest. *J. Agric. Food Chem.* **2008**, *56*, 11447–11452. [CrossRef] [PubMed]
23. Kolayli, S.; Sahin, H.; Can, Z.; Yildiz, O.; Malkoc, M.; Asadov, A. A member of complementary medicinal food: anatolian royal jellies, their chemical compositions, and antioxidant properties. *J. Evid. Based Complement. Altern. Med.* **2016**, *21*, NP43–NP48. [CrossRef] [PubMed]
24. Yang, Y.C.; Chou, W.M.; Widowati, D.A.; Lin, I.P.; Peng, C.C. 10-hydroxy-2-decenoic acid of royal jelly exhibits bactericide and anti-inflammatory activity in human colon cancer cells. *BMC Complement. Altern. Med.* **2018**, *18*, 202. [CrossRef] [PubMed]
25. Hajra, S.; Patra, A.R.; Basu, A.; Bhattacharya, S. Prevention of doxorubicin (DOX)-induced genotoxicity and cardiotoxicity: Effect of plant derived small molecule indole-3-carbinol (I3C) on oxidative stress and inflammation. *Biomed. Pharmacother.* **2018**, *101*, 228–243. [CrossRef] [PubMed]
26. Pugazhendhi, A.; Edison, T.N.J.I.; Velmurugan, B.K.; Jacob, J.A.; Karuppusamy, I. Toxicity of Doxorubicin (Dox) to different experimental organ systems. *Life Sci.* **2018**, *200*, 26–30. [CrossRef] [PubMed]
27. Kaynar, L.; Cetin, A.; Hacioglu, S.K.; Eser, B.; Koçyigit, İ.; Canöz, Ö.; Tasdemir, A.; Karadag, C.; Kurnaz, F.; Saraymen, R.; et al. Efficacy of royal jelly on methotrexate-induced systemic oxidative stress and damage to small intestine in rats. *Afr. J. Tradit. Complement. Altern. Med.* **2012**, *9*, 412–417. [CrossRef] [PubMed]
28. Suemaru, K.; Cui, R.; Li, B.; Watanabe, S.; Okihara, K.; Hashimoto, K.; Yamada, H.; Araki, H. Topical application of royal jelly has a healing effect for 5-fluorouracil-induced experimental oral mucositis in hamsters. *Methods Find. Exp. Clin. Pharmacol.* **2008**, *30*, 103–106. [CrossRef]
29. Karadeniz, A.; Simsek, N.; Karakus, E.; Yildirim, S.; Kara, A.; Can, I.; Kisa, F.; Emre, H.; Turkeli, M. Royal jelly modulates oxidative stress and apoptosis in liver and kidneys of rats treated with cisplatin. *Oxid. Med. Cell. Longev.* **2011**, *2011*, 981793. [CrossRef]
30. Ibrahim, A.; Eldaim, M.A.; Abdel-Daim, M.M. Nephroprotective effect of bee honey and royal jelly against subchronic cisplatin toxicity in rats. *Cytotechnology* **2016**, *68*, 1039–1048. [CrossRef]
31. Erdem, O.; Güngörmüş, Z. The effect of royal jelly on oral mucositis in patients undergoing radiotherapy and chemotherapy. *Holist. Nurs. Pract.* **2014**, *28*, 242–246. [CrossRef] [PubMed]
32. Yamauchi, K.; Kogashiwa, Y.; Moro, Y.; Kohno, N. The effect of topical application of royal jelly on chemoradiotherapy-induced mucositis in head and neck cancer: A preliminary study. *Int. J. Otolaryngol.* **2014**, *2014*, 974967. [CrossRef]
33. Mofid, B.; Rezaeizadeh, H.; Termos, A.; Rakhsha, A.; Mafi, A.R.; Taheripanah, T.; Ardakani, M.M.; Taghavi, S.M.; Moravveji, S.A.; Kashi, A.S. Effect of processed honey and royal jelly on cancer-related fatigue: A double-blind randomized clinical trial. *Electron Phys.* **2016**, *8*, 2475–2482. [CrossRef] [PubMed]

34. Osama, H.; Abdullah, A.; Gamal, B.; Emad, D.; Sayed, D.; Hussein, E.; Mahfouz, E.; Tharwat, J.; Sayed, S.; Medhat, S.; et al. Effect of honey and royal jelly against cisplatin-induced nephrotoxicity in patients with cancer. *J. Am. Coll. Nutr.* **2017**, *36*, 342–346. [CrossRef] [PubMed]
35. Miyata, Y.; Matsuo, T.; Araki, K.; Nakamura, Y.; Sagara, Y.; Ohba, K.; Sakai, H. Anticancer effects of green tea and the underlying molecular mechanisms in bladder cancer. *Medicines (Basel)* **2018**, *5*, 87. [CrossRef]
36. Ohba, K.; Miyata, Y.; Watanabe, S.; Hayashi, T.; Kanetake, H.; Kanda, S.; Sakai, H. Clinical significance and predictive value of prostaglandin E2 receptors (EPR) 1–4 in patients with renal cell carcinoma. *Anticancer Res.* **2011**, *31*, 597–605.
37. Silici, S.; Ekmekcioglu, O.; Kanbur, M.; Deniz, K. The protective effect of royal jelly against cisplatin-induced renal oxidative stress in rats. *World J. Urol.* **2011**, *29*, 127–132. [CrossRef]
38. Yamaura, K.; Tomono, A.; Suwa, E.; Ueno, K. Topical royal jelly alleviates symptoms of pruritus in a murine model of allergic contact dermatitis. *Pharmacogn. Mag.* **2013**, *9*, 9–13. [CrossRef]
39. Khazaei, M.; Ansarian, A.; Ghanbari, E. New findings on biological actions and clinical applications of royal jelly: A review. *J. Diet. Suppl.* **2018**, *15*, 757–775. [CrossRef]
40. Kamakura, M.; Mitani, N.; Fukuda, T.; Fukushima, M. Antifatigue effect of fresh royal jelly in mice. *J. Nutr. Sci. Vitaminol. (Tokyo)* **2001**, *47*, 394–401. [CrossRef]
41. Del Fabbro, E. Current and future care of patients with the cancer anorexia-cachexia syndrome. *Am. Soc. Clin. Oncol. Educ. Book* **2015**, e229–e237. [CrossRef] [PubMed]
42. Macciò, A.; Madeddu, C.; Mantovani, G. Current pharmacotherapy options for cancer anorexia and cachexia. *Expert Opin. Pharmacother.* **2012**, *13*, 2453–2472. [CrossRef] [PubMed]
43. Fujiwara, S.; Imai, J.; Fujiwara, M.; Yaeshima, T.; Kawashima, T.; Kobayashi, K. A potent antibacterial protein in royal jelly. Purification and determination of the primary structure of royalisin. *J. Biol. Chem.* **1990**, *265*, 11333–11337. [PubMed]
44. Watanabe, K.; Shinmoto, H.; Kobori, M.; Tsushida, T.; Shinohara, K.; Kanaeda, J.; Yonekura, M. Stimulation of cell growth in the U-937 human myeloid cell line by honey royal jelly protein. *Cytotechnology* **1998**, *26*, 23–27. [CrossRef] [PubMed]
45. Honda, Y.; Araki, Y.; Hata, T.; Ichihara, K.; Ito, M.; Tanaka, M.; Honda, S. 10-Hydroxy-2-decenoic acid, the major Lipid component of royal jelly, extends the lifespan of caenorhabditis elegans through dietary restriction and target of rapamycin signaling. *J. Aging Res.* **2015**, *2015*, 425261. [CrossRef] [PubMed]

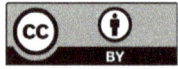

© 2018 by the authors. Licensee MDPI, Basel, Switzerland. This article is an open access article distributed under the terms and conditions of the Creative Commons Attribution (CC BY) license (http://creativecommons.org/licenses/by/4.0/).

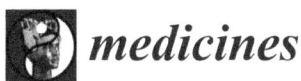

Article

Bioactive Composition, Antioxidant Activity, and Anticancer Potential of Freeze-Dried Extracts from Defatted Gac (*Momordica cochinchinensis* Spreng) Seeds

Anh V. Le [1,2,*], Tien T. Huynh [3], Sophie E. Parks [1,4], Minh H. Nguyen [1,5] and Paul D. Roach [1]

1. School of Environmental and Life Sciences, University of Newcastle, Ourimbah, NSW 2258, Australia; sophie.parks@dpi.nsw.gov.au (S.E.P.); Minh.Nguyen@newcastle.edu.au (M.H.N.); Paul.Roach@newcastle.edu.au (P.D.R.)
2. Faculty of Bio-Food Technology and Environment, University of Technology (HUTECH), Ho Chi Minh City 700000, Vietnam
3. School of Science, RMIT University, Bundoora, VIC 3083, Australia; tien.huynh@rmit.edu.au
4. Central Coast Primary Industries Centre, NSW Department of Primary Industries, Ourimbah, NSW 2258, Australia
5. School of Science and Health, Western Sydney University, Penrith, NSW 2751, Australia
* Correspondence: vananh.le@uon.edu.au

Received: 6 September 2018; Accepted: 15 September 2018; Published: 18 September 2018

Abstract: Background: Gac (*Momordica cochinchinensis* Spreng) seeds have long been used in traditional medicine as a remedy for numerous conditions due to a range of bioactive compounds. This study investigated the solvent extraction of compounds that could be responsible for antioxidant activity and anticancer potential. **Methods:** Defatted Gac seed kernel powder was extracted with different solvents: 100% water, 50% methanol:water, 70% ethanol:water, water saturated butanol, 100% methanol, and 100% ethanol. Trypsin inhibitors, saponins, phenolics, and antioxidant activity using the 2,2'-azino-bis(3-ethylbenzothiazoline-6-sulfonic acid) diammonium salt (ABTS), the 2,2-diphenyl-1-picrylhydrazyl (DPPH) and the ferric reducing antioxidant power (FRAP) assays; and anticancer potential against two melanoma cancer cell lines (MM418C1 and D24) were analysed to determine the best extraction solvents. **Results:** Water was best for extracting trypsin inhibitors (581.4 ± 18.5 mg trypsin/mg) and reducing the viability of MM418C1 and D24 melanoma cells (75.5 ± 1.3 and 66.9 ± 2.2%, respectively); the anticancer potential against the MM418C1 cells was highly correlated with trypsin inhibitors ($r = 0.92$, $p < 0.05$), but there was no correlation between anticancer potential and antioxidant activity. The water saturated butanol had the highest saponins (71.8 ± 4.31 mg aescin equivalents/g), phenolic compounds (20.4 ± 0.86 mg gallic acid equivalents/g), and antioxidant activity, but these measures were not related to anticancer potential. **Conclusions:** Water yielded a Gac seed extract, rich in trypsin inhibitors, which had high anticancer potential against two melanoma cell lines.

Keywords: *Momordica cochinchinensis*; Gac; seeds; saponins; trypsin inhibitors; phenolics; anticancer; antioxidant; extraction; freeze dried extract

---

1. Introduction

Momordica cochinchinensis Spreng, commonly called Gac, is a plant species of the family Cucurbitaceae, which is also known as red melon, baby jackfruit, spiny bitter gourd, sweet gourd, and cochinchin gourd. It is native to Southeast Asia and is commonly grown as a food crop in Vietnam, Thailand, Laos, Myanmar, and Cambodia [1,2]. From the food and commercial perspectives, the most commonly used part of the mature fruit is the red flesh surrounding the seeds, called the aril, which is traditionally used as a colourant in rice or, more recently, as a material that is processed into functional food ingredients or supplements [3].

The seeds are not eaten; they are removed from the aril and are mostly considered as waste [3,4]. However, in traditional medicine, Gac seeds are purported to have an array of therapeutic effects on a variety of conditions, such as fluxes, liver and spleen disorders, haemorrhoids, wounds, bruises, swelling, and pus [2,5]. In modern research, several constituents have been identified, which could be involved in the putative medicinal properties of Gac seeds, including trypsin inhibitors (e.g., MCoTI-I, MCoTI-II and MCoTI-III) [6–8], saponins (e.g., Momordica Saponin I and Momordica Saponin II) [9,10], and phenolic compounds (e.g., gallic acid and *p*-hydroxybenzoic acid) [11]. Gac seed extracts have been linked with many medicinal properties, such as gastroprotective [12–14], anti-inflammatory [15,16], anticancer [17], and antitumor [18] activities. Most of these properties are linked to the seed's saponins [12,13,15,16]. Furthermore, karounidiol, a triterpenoid compound, likely a saponin, present in Gac seeds [19], possess cytotoxic activity against human cancer cell lines [20]. Protease inhibitors, like the trypsin inhibitors in Gac seeds [7,8,21], have diverse biochemical functions [4,22], including acting as anticancer agents by inhibiting the growth of transformed cells [23–26]. Some trypsin inhibitors, such as those from *Cajanus cajan* and *Phaseolus limensis*, possess antioxidant, anti-inflammatory, and anti-bacterial activity [27].

There is limited information on how to best recover the bioactive compounds from Gac seeds, particularly to optimise anticancer potential. Efficient extraction and preservation methods are important for their immediate and long-term use. For any given plant bioactive, extractable yield depends on the extraction solvent, the chemical nature of the targeted component, and the characteristics of the extraction procedure. When other factors are kept constant, the extraction solvent plays a key role in obtaining the desired quality and quantity of the target constituents [28,29]. The choice of solvent is mainly based on the chemical properties of the targeted compounds, such as their polarity or hydrophobicity.

Due to the hydrophilic or amphiphilic nature of the trypsin inhibitors, phenolics, and saponins in Gac seeds, aqueous solvents and the low alcohols are likely to be the best extraction solvents for these bioactive compounds. They are also the safest and the most environmentally-friendly solvents for the extraction of bioactive compounds from plant materials [30,31]. For drying after solvent extractions, numerous methods have been developed; however, freeze drying is considered to be superior for preserving the medicinal qualities of botanical extracts and it is therefore widely used [32]. Additionally, to make it easier for the extraction of trypsin inhibitors [33] and to avoid interference of sticky oil during the freeze-drying procedure, the Gac seeds need to be defatted before they are extracted with solvents.

Thus, this study aimed to investigate the effectiveness of different solvents (water, alcohols, and mixtures) to extract the bioactive compounds of interest (trypsin inhibitors, saponins, and phenolics) from defatted Gac seed kernel powder. The relationships between the extracted compounds and the antioxidant activity and the anticancer potential of the extracts were also investigated.

2. Materials and Methods

2.1. Materials

2.1.1. Solvents, Reagents, and Chemicals

Solvents (ethanol, methanol and butanol) and chemicals (vanillin, sulphuric acid and potassium persulfate) were purchased from Merck (Bayswater, VIC, Australia). Folin-ciocalteu's phenol reagent, anhydrous sodium carbonate, sodium nitrile, ferric chloride, gallic acid, catechin, 2,4,6-tris(2-pyridyl)-s-triazine, (±)-6-hydroxy-2,5,7,8-tetramethylchromane-2-carboxylic acid (trolox), aescin, 2,2-diphenyl-1-picrylhydrazyl (DPPH), 2,2′-azino-bis(3-ethylbenzothiazoline-6-sulfonic acid) diammonium salt (ABTS), trypsin (type I) from bovine pancreas, benzyl-DL-arginine-para-nitroanilide

(BAPNA), Tris, and dimethylsulfoxide (DMSO) were purchased from Sigma-Aldrich Co. (Castle Hill, NSW, Australia). Sodium acetate trihydrate was purchased from Government Stores Department (Sydney, NSW, Australia). Aluminium chloride was a product of J. T. Baker Chem. Co. (Thermo Fisher Scientific, North Ryde, NSW, Australia). Acetic acid was a product of BDH Laboratory Supplies (Bio-Strategy, Tingalpa, QLD, Australia). Sodium hydroxide was a product of Ajax FineChem (Thermo Fisher Scientific, North Ryde, NSW, Australia) and hydrochloride acid a product of Lab-Scan Ltd. (Bacto, Mt Pritchard, NSW, Australia).

Human melanoma MM418C1 (mutated BRAF oncogene), referred to as C1 melanoma cells, and D24 (wild type BRAF oncogene) and human keratinocyte (HaCat) cell lines were provided by the School of Health and Biomedical Sciences, RMIT University (Bundoora, VIC, Australia). RPMI-1640 media, streptomycin, and penicillin were Gibco products (Thermo Fisher Scientific, North Ryde, NSW, Australia). Fetal bovine serum (FBS) was from Serana (Melbourne, VIC, Australia).

2.1.2. Gac Seeds

Gac seeds, from accession VS7 as classified by Wimalasiri et al. [1], were collected from 450 kg of fresh Gac fruit. These fruits were bought at Gac fruit fields in Dong Nai province, Ho Chi Minh City, Vietnam (Latitude: 10.757410; Longitude: 106.673439). After their separation from the fresh fruit, the seeds were vacuum dried at 40 °C for 24 h to reduce moisture and increase the crispness of the shell, which facilitated shell removal. The dried seeds were de-coated to get the kernels, which were then packaged in vacuum-sealed aluminium bags and stored at -18 °C until used.

Preparation of Defatted Gac Seed Kernel Powder

Defatted Gac seed kernel powder was prepared as described by Le et al. [34]. Briefly, the Gac seed kernels were ground in an electric grinder (100 g ST-02A Mulry Disintegrator, Taiwan Machinary, Sydney, NSW, Australia) to a powder that could pass through a sieve of 1.4 mm. The powder was then freeze-dried using a Dynavac FD3 Freeze Dryer (Dynapumps, Seven Hills, NSW, Australia) for 48 h, at -45 °C under vacuum at a pressure loading of 10^{-2} mbar (1 Pa), to reduce the moisture content to $1.21 \pm 0.02\%$. The powder was then defatted using three 30-min extractions with hexane at a powder to hexane ratio of 1:5 w/v. The resulting slurry was suction filtered and the residue (defatted meal) was air-dried for 12 h and stored in a desiccator at ambient room temperature until used. The moisture content of the defatted powder, measured using a Shimadzu MOC63u moisture analyser (Rydalmere, NSW, Australia), was $8.61 \pm 0.15\%$.

2.2. Methods

2.2.1. Extraction

Based on a previous study [34], six solvents (deionised water, 100% methanol, 50% methanol in water, 100% ethanol, 70% ethanol in water, and 90% n-butanol in water), were used for the extraction of bioactive compounds from the defatted and dried Gac seed kernel powder. Twenty grams of the powder were added to 400 mL of each solvent and the suspension was kept under constant magnetic stirring for 30 min at 40 ± 1 °C. Following extraction, the mixtures were filtered through two layers of cheese cloth and then through a Whatman No. 1 filter paper (Thermo Fisher Scientific, North Ryde, NSW, Australia), and the clear filtrates were collected in 500 mL evaporating flasks. Triplicate extractions were done for each solvent.

2.2.2. Freeze Drying Extracts

The filtrates collected from the extractions were freeze-dried into powders as summarized in Figure 1. First, the liquid extracts were concentrated using a rotary evaporator (Buchi Rotavapor B480, Buchi Australia, Noble Park, VIC, Australia) at 40 °C under vacuum until thick but not completely dried in the 500 mL evaporating flasks. Then, to transfer the extracts into pre-weighed 100 mL evaporating flasks, three different solvents were used. For each of the butanol, methanol, and 50% methanol extracts, 50 mL of 50% methanol in water was used, for each of the ethanol and 70% ethanol extracts, 50 mL of 50% ethanol in water was used, and for the water extract, 30 mL of water was used. The suspensions were mixed well, and the evaporation resumed until around 20 mL of the concentrated extracts were left. The concentrates were then frozen using liquid nitrogen before freeze drying with a BenchTop Pro freeze dryer (Scitek, Lane Cove, NSW, Australia) at −60 °C and 30 mbar for 48 h. The flasks with residue were placed in a desiccator and quickly weighed. The difference in weight between the flasks with residue and the empty flasks was taken to be the mass recovered for each extract. These freeze dried (FD) crude extracts were then stored in air-tight containers at −20 °C for use within 3 months.

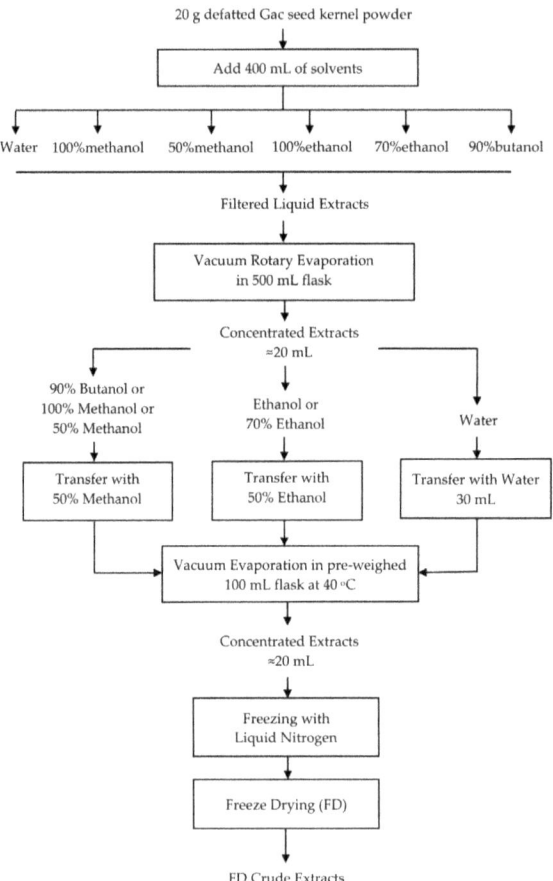

Figure 1. Procedure for producing freeze dried (FD) crude extracts from defatted Gac seed kernel powder.

2.2.3. Determination of Extractable Yield

To determine the extractable yield, 10 mL of each filtered liquid extract, resulting from Section 2.2.1, was transferred into a tared flat-bottomed glass vial and then dried at 105 °C with a vacuum pressure of 60 kPa for 24 h in a vacuum oven (Thermoline, Wetherill Park, NSW, Australia) until a constant weight was achieved. These vials were cooled in a desiccator for 30 min and weighed. The extractable yield was calculated, in g dried extract per 100 g of dried defatted Gac seed kernel powder, using Equation (1), where EY was the extractable yield, DE (g) was the mass of dried extract after the vacuum oven drying,

40 was the ratio of the 10 mL used for the vacuum oven drying to the 400 mL originally used for the extract, and DS (g) was the mass of dried defatted Gac seed kernel powder used for the extraction.

$$\text{EY (g/100 g)} = \frac{\text{DE} \times 40}{\text{DS}} \times 100 \tag{1}$$

2.2.4. Determination of Dry Mass Yield

Dry mass yield was defined as the amount (g) of FD crude extract, produced as described in Section 2.2.2, per 100 g of dried defatted Gac seed kernel powder. Equation (2) was used to calculate the dry mass yield (DM), in which FD (g) was the weight of the FD crude extract, DS (g) was the mass of dried defatted Gac seed kernel powder used for the extraction, and V was the volume of the filtrate collected after extraction.

$$\text{DM (g/100 g)} = \frac{\text{FD} \times V/(V-10)}{\text{DS}} \times 100 \tag{2}$$

2.2.5. Determination of Trypsin Inhibitor Activity (TIA)

The TIA assay was performed as described by Makkar et al. [35] except that the absorbance was measured at 385 nm, as suggested by Stauffer [36], instead of at 410 nm.

Reagent Preparation

Substrate solution: A substrate solution of 92 mM BAPNA was prepared as follows. First, 40.0 mg BAPNA was dissolved in 1.00 mL DMSO and diluted to 100 mL with 0.05 M Tris-buffer (pH 8.2) containing 0.02 M $CaCl_2$ pre-warmed to 37 °C. This solution was prepared daily and kept at 37 °C while in use.

Trypsin solution: 20.0 mg of trypsin (type I) from bovine pancreas was dissolved in 1 mM HCl to make 1 L and stored at 4 °C for use within a week. In the analytical procedure with 92 mM BAPNA, this solution gave an absorbance value in the range of 0.900 ± 0.010 after subtracting the reagent blank at 385 nm.

Determination of TIA

Each FD crude extract from Section 2.2.2 (Figure 1) was dissolved in water at a concentration to give an inhibition of Trypsin between 40% and 60% and the assay was setup as shown in Table 1 with four test tubes prepared for each FD crude extract. All the prepared test tubes were kept in a water bath at 37 °C for 10 min to promote the formation of an enzyme–inhibitor complex and then 5.0 mL of BAPNA solution, pre-warmed to 37 °C, was added into each tube and the tubes were incubated in a water bath at 37 °C for 10 min. One mL of 30% acetic acid solution was added to each tube to stop the reaction. Then, 2.0 mL of trypsin solution was added into each reagent and sample blank (Table 1). After thorough mixing, the absorbance of the reaction mixture due to the release of p–nitroaniline was measured at 385 nm.

Table 1. The trypsin inhibitor activity assay setup.

Component	Reagent Blank (a)	Standard (b)	Sample Blank (c)	Sample (d)
Deionised water (mL)	2	2	1	1
Trypsin solution (mL)	-	2	-	2
Diluted extract (mL)	-	-	1	1
BAPNA (mL)	5	5	5	5
Acetic acid (mL)	1	1	1	1
Trypsin solution after reaction inactivation (mL)	2	-	2	-

BAPNA (benzyl-DL-arginine-para-nitroanilide) was added to start the reaction and acetic acid for inactivation.

Calculation

The change in absorbance (A_I) due to the trypsin inhibitor per mL of diluted extract was ($A_b - A_a$) − ($A_d - A_c$), where the subscripts referred to tubes (a) to (d) in Table 1. Since 1 µg of trypsin gave an absorbance of 0.0190, the weight of trypsin inhibited per mL of extract was $A_I/0.019$ µg. From this value, The TIA of the FD crude extracts was calculated using Equation (3) and expressed as mg of pure trypsin inhibited per mg of FD crude extract.

$$TIA = \frac{A_I}{0.019 \times S \times \left(1 - \frac{m\%}{100}\right)} \quad (3)$$

where,

A_I: Change in absorbance due to inhibition per 1 mL of extract;
$A_I = (A_b - A_a) - (A_d - A_c)$, subscripts as per Table 1;
S: Weight (mg) of the FD crude extract dissolved in 1 mL;
m%: Moisture content of the FD crude extract powder.

2.2.6. Determination of Total Saponin Content (TSC)

The FD crude extracts from Section 2.2.2 were dissolved in water at a concentration of 2 mg/mL and vortexed before the TSC was determined according to Tan et al. [37] with some modifications. Briefly, 0.25 mL of each extract was mixed with 0.25 mL of 8% (w/v) vanillin solution and 2.5 mL of 72% (v/v) sulphuric acid. The mixture was vortexed and incubated in a water bath at 60 °C for 15 min and then cooled on ice for 10 min. The absorption of the mixture was measured at 560 nm using a Cary 60 UV-Vis spectrophotometer (Agilent Technologies, Mulgrave, VIC, Australia). Aecsin was used as a standard and the results were expressed as milligram aecsin equivalents (AE) per gram of the FD crude extract powder (mg AE/g).

2.2.7. Determination of Total Phenolic Content (TPC)

The FD crude extracts from Section 2.2.2 were dissolved in water at a concentration of 2 mg/mL and vortexed before the TPC was determined according to the method of Tan et al. [38] with some modifications. Briefly, 0.5 mL of each extract was mixed with 2.5 mL of 10% (v/v) Folin–Ciocalteu reagent in water and incubated at room temperature for 2 min to equilibrate. Then, 2 mL of 7.5% (w/v) sodium carbonate solution in water was added and the mixture was incubated at ambient temperature for 1 h. The absorption of the reaction mixture was measured at 765 nm using a Cary 60 UV-Vis spectrophotometer. Gallic acid was used as a standard and the results were expressed as milligram gallic acid equivalents (GAE) per gram dry weight of the FD crude extract powder (mg GAE/g).

2.2.8. Determination of Antioxidant Capacity

The FD crude extracts from Section 2.2.2 were dissolved in water at the concentration of 2 mg/mL and mixed before analysing antioxidant capacity using three assays: the 2,2'-azino-bis(3-ethylbenzothiazoline-6-sulfonic acid) diammonium salt (ABTS), the 2,2-diphenyl-1-picrylhydrazyl (DPPH) and the ferric reducing antioxidant power (FRAP).

DPPH

The DPPH assay measures the total free radical scavenging capacity of the extracts. The assay was performed as described by Tan et al. [38]. A stock solution of 0.6 M DPPH in methanol was prepared and kept at −20 °C until use. The working solution was prepared by mixing 10 mL of stock solution with 45 mL of methanol to obtain an absorbance of 1.1 ± 0.02 units at 515 nm using a spectrophotometer. Each extract (0.15 mL) was mixed with 2.85 mL of the working solution and the mixture was allowed to stand for 3 h, after which the absorption was measured at 515 nm using a

Cary 60 UV-Vis spectrophotometer. Trolox was used as a standard and the results were expressed as milligram Trolox equivalents (TE) per gram of the FD crude extract powder (mg TE/g).

ABTS

The ABTS assay measures the total free radical scavenging capacity of the extracts. The assay was performed as described by Tan et al. [38] with slight modifications. Stock solutions of 7.4 mM ABTS and 2.6 mM potassium persulfate were freshly prepared or kept at 4 °C in a dark bottle for use within a month, respectively. A fresh working solution was prepared for each assay by mixing equal quantities of the two stock solutions and incubated for 15 h to 16 h in the dark at ambient temperature. Then, 1 mL of the working solution was diluted with approximately 30 mL of methanol to obtain an absorbance of 1.1 ± 0.02 units at 734 nm using a Cary 60 UV-Vis spectrophotometer. Each extract (0.15 mL) was mixed with 2.85 mL of the working solution and the mixture was incubated for 2 h in the dark at ambient temperature. The absorption of the reaction mixture was measured at 734 nm using a Cary 60 UV-Vis spectrophotometer. Trolox was used as a standard and the results were expressed as milligram Trolox equivalents (TE) per gram of the FD crude extract powder (mg TE/g).

FRAP

The FRAP assay measures the ferric reducing power. The assay was performed following the method of Thaipong et al. [39], based on the increase in absorbance at 593 nm. A fresh FRAP working solution was initially prepared by mixing 300 mM acetate buffer (pH 3.6), 10 mM iron reagent (TPTZ) in 40 mM HCl, and 20 mM $FeCl_3 \bullet 6H_2O$ in the ratio of 10:1:1 ($v/v/v$). The fresh working solution was warmed to 37 °C before using. Each extract (0.15 mL) was mixed with 2.85 mL of the working FRAP solution and the mixture was incubated at ambient temperature in the dark for 30 min before its absorbance was measured at 593 nm using a Cary 60 UV-Vis spectrophotometer. Trolox was used as a standard and the antioxidant capacity of each sample, based on its ability to reduce ferric ions, was expressed as milligram Trolox equivalents (TE) per gram of the FD crude extract powder (mg TE/g).

2.2.9. Determination of Cytotoxicity

Cell Lines and Culture

The human melanoma MM418C1 (C1, wild type BRAF oncogene) and D24 (mutated BRAF oncogene) cell lines were maintained in RPMI-1640 media supplemented with 10% (v/v) FBS, 1% (v/v) streptomycin and penicillin at 37 °C in 5% CO_2. HaCat keratinocytes were used as normal untransformed cells and grown in the same media.

In Vitro Cytotoxicity Assay

All cells were seeded in 96 well plates (Greiner Bio-One, Labfriend, Sydney, NSW, Australia), 5000 cells/well along with 100 µL of fresh media. The FD crude extracts from Section 2.2.2 were dissolved in RPMI-1640 cell culture media at a concentration of 2 mg/mL and UV-sterilised for 10 min in a laminar flow hood before use on cells. The cells were allowed to attach for 4 h before being treated with 10 µL of the extract and incubated for 48 h.

The effect of the extracts on cell growth was determined using the CCK-8 (Cell Counting Kit-8) assay (Sigma-Aldrich, St Louis, MO, USA). The assay measured cytotoxicity based on the conversion of a water-soluble tetrazolium salt, 2-(2-methoxy-4-nitrophenyl)-3-(4-nitrophenyl)-5-(2,4-disulfophenyl)-2H-tetrazolium, monosodium salt (WST-8), to a water-soluble formazan dye upon reduction by dehydrogenases in the presence of an electron carrier [40].

To determine cell viability, 10 µL of CCK-8 solution was added to each well of the 96-well plate containing treated and control samples. The plates were incubated at 37 °C for 2 h and the absorbance was measured spectrophotometrically at 450 nm using a CLARIOstar® High Performance Monochromator Multimode Microplate Reader (BMG LABTECH, Mornington, NSW, Australia) and the results were analysed using the MARS data analysis software (version 3.00R2, BMG LABTECH, Mornington, NSW, Australia). The data were presented as a proportional viability (%) by comparing the treated cells with the untreated cells (control) using Equation (4):

$$\text{Cell viability} = \frac{At - Ab}{Ac - Ab} \times 100 \qquad (4)$$

where At was the absorbance value of the treated cells, Ab was the absorbance of CCK-8 only, and Ac was the negative control which included cells and CCK-8 only. Two types of controls were used: the media control consisted of cultured cells in 10% (v/v) FBS containing medium alone and the vehicle control consisted of cells in 10% (v/v) FBS containing medium, to which 10 µL of RPMI-1640 media without FBS was added. However, as both controls did not cause cytotoxicity, the media control was used to calculate cell viability.

Cell morphology was analysed at 48 h using a Nikon Eclipse TS100 (Nikon, Tokyo, Japan) phase contrast inverted microscope and the images were captured using a Nikon DS-Fi1digital camera.

2.2.10. Statistical Analyses

Extractions were performed in triplicate and means ± standard deviation (SD) were assessed with the one-way Analysis of Variance (ANOVA) and Tukey's *Post Hoc* Multiple Comparisons test using the IBM SPSS Statistics 24 program (IBM Corp., Armonk, NY, USA). Differences in means were considered statistically significant at $p < 0.05$. Correlations and their significance were determined using the Microsoft Excel 2016 (Microsoft Corp., Seattle, WA, USA) and Principle Component Analysis (Minitab 17.1.0, Sydney, NSW, Australia).

3. Results

3.1. Effect of Solvent on the Extractable Yield and the Dry Mass Yield

Extractable yield and dry mass yield were calculated for each extract. The extractable yields ranged from 4.4 g/100 g for the ethanol extract to 15.5 g/100 g for the aqueous extract while the dry mass yield ranged from 3.7 g/100 g for the ethanol extract to 13.1 g/100 g for the aqueous extract (Table 2). For both the extractable yield and the dry mass yield, the values were substantially higher for the aqueous extracts than for the organic solvents, whether they were mixed with water or not. Furthermore, the extractable yield (before drying) was higher than the dry mass yield (after freeze drying) for all extracts. The observed loss during the drying process was highest for the 70% ethanol extract (−31%) followed by the methanol extract (−28%) and the butanol extract (−20%). The aqueous and ethanol extracts had the same loss (−15%), while the lowest lost was for the 50% methanol extract (−11%).

Table 2. Effect of solvent on the extractable yield (EY) and the dry mass yield (DM).

Solvent	EY (g/100 g)	DM (g/100 g)	Original Volume (mL)	Collected Volume (mL)	Yield Loss (%)
Water	15.5 ± 0.1 [a]	13.1 ± 0.1 [b]	400 ± 3	355 ± 0	15.3 ± 0.1 [d]
50% Methanol	10.2 ± 0.0 [c]	9.1 ± 0.3 [d]	400 ± 3	348 ± 3	10.9 ± 0.2 [f]
70% Ethanol	10.2 ± 0.0 [c]	7.1 ± 0.4 [e]	400 ± 3	340 ± 5	30.6 ± 0.3 [a]
90% Butanol	6.9 ± 0.1 [e]	5.5 ± 0.1 [f]	400 ± 3	350 ± 0	19.9 ± 0.1 [c]
Methanol	6.7 ± 0.2 [e]	4.8 ± 0.2 [g]	400 ± 3	330 ± 0	27.8 ± 0.2 [b]
Ethanol	4.4 ± 0.0 [g]	3.7 ± 0.0 [h]	400 ± 3	345 ± 0	14.9 ± 0.0 [e]

The values were the means ± SD of three replicate extractions for each solvent. All the values for EY and DM were compared to each other, the values for yield loss were compared separately and the values not sharing the same superscript letter for EY and DM, and separately for yield loss, were significantly different at $p < 0.05$.

3.2. Effect of Solvents on the Content of Bioactive Compounds

3.2.1. Trypsin Inhibitors

The yield of trypsin inhibitors was measured as the trypsin inhibitor activity (TIA) of the FD crude extracts (Figure 2). The water extract had the highest TIA (581.4 mg/mg) and the yield decreased relative to the concentration of water in the water and low alcohol mixtures: −40% for the 50% methanol (≈50% water) extract, −54% for the 70% ethanol (≈30% water) extract and −97% for the water-saturated butanol (≈10% water) extract. The 100% methanol and 100% ethanol extracts had much lower TIA values than the water extract, −96% and −95%, respectively (Figure 2). Therefore, water was the best solvent for extracting trypsin inhibitors from the defatted Gac seed kernel powder.

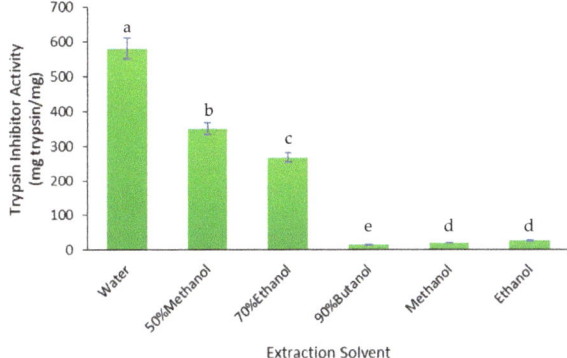

Figure 2. Effect of solvent on the trypsin inhibitor activity (TIA) of the FD crude extracts. The values are the means ± SD of three replicate extractions for each solvent. Columns not sharing the same letter are significantly different at $p < 0.05$.

3.2.2. Saponins

The yield of saponins was measured as the total saponin content (TSC) of the FD crude extracts (Figure 3). The highest TSC was found in the butanol and methanol extracts, which were 24% higher than the TSC in the 50% methanol and 70% ethanol extracts, 48% higher than the ethanol extract, and 53% higher than the water extract. Therefore, butanol and methanol were the best solvents for extracting the saponins from the defatted Gac seed kernel powder.

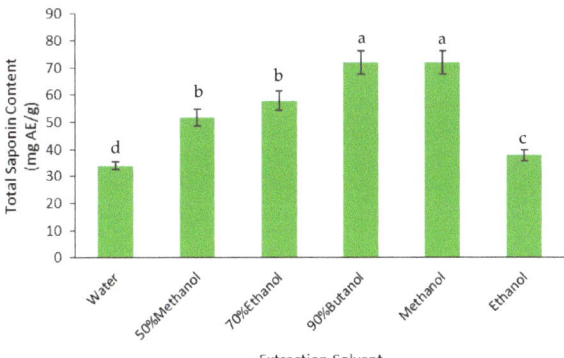

Figure 3. Effect of solvent on the total saponin content (TSC) extraction from Gac seed. The values were the means ± SD of three replicate extractions for each solvent. Columns not sharing the same letter were significantly different at $p < 0.05$.

3.2.3. Phenolics

The yield of phenolics was measured as the total phenolic content (TPC) of the FD crude extracts (Figure 4). The highest TPC was found in the butanol extract; the TPC in this extract was 13% higher than the water extract, 29% higher than the 50% methanol and 70% ethanol extracts, 35% higher than the methanol extract, and 63% higher than the ethanol extract. Therefore, butanol extracted the highest phenolics from the defatted Gac seed kernel powder.

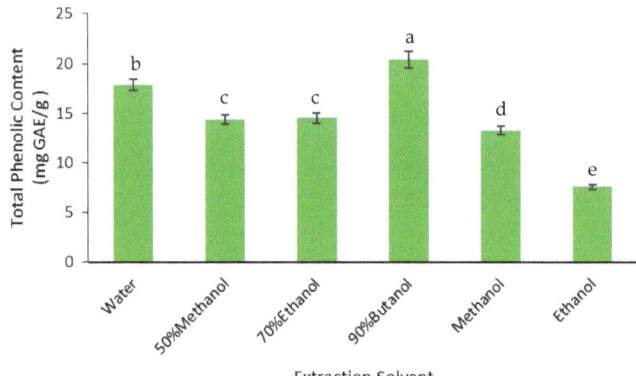

Figure 4. Effect of solvent on the total phenolic content (TPC) of the FD Gac seed crude extracts. The values were the means ± SD of three replicate extractions for each solvent. Columns not sharing the same letter were significantly different at $p < 0.05$. GAE, Gallic acid equivalents.

3.3. Effect of Solvents on Antioxidant Activity

The antioxidant activity of the extracts was measured using three assays: DPPH, ABTS, and FRAP. The butanol extract gave the highest values for ABTS and DPPH assays and the ethanol extract gave the highest value for FRAP assay (Figure 5). These two extracts produced significantly higher antioxidant activity based on the ABTS, DPPH, and FRAP assays (Figure 5).

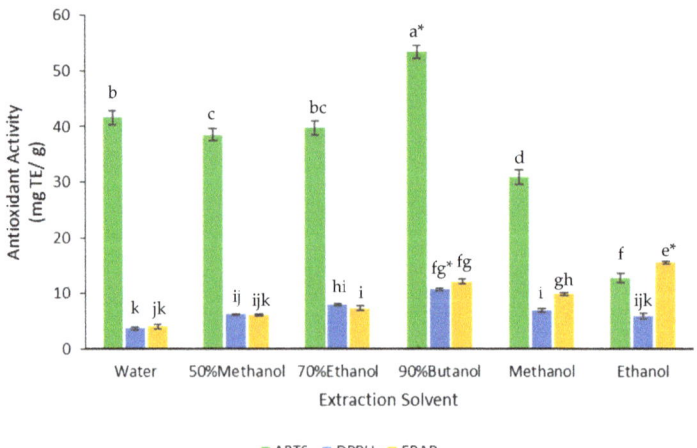

Figure 5. Effect of solvent on the antioxidant capacity of the FD crude extracts. The values were the means ± SD of three replicate extractions for each solvent. Columns not sharing the same superscript letter were significantly different at $p < 0.05$. * indicated the highest antioxidant activity. TE, Trolox equivalents.

3.4. Effect of Extraction Solvent on Cancer Cell Viability

The FD crude extracts were tested for cell toxicity using two melanoma cell lines (D24 and C1) and a normal keratinocyte line (HaCat). The water extract was the most cytotoxic towards both cancer cell lines compared to the other extracts (Figure 6); the extract decreased the cell viability by 67% for D24 and 75% for C1 melanoma cells. The 70% ethanol and 50% methanol extracts also showed cytotoxic activity towards the C1 melanoma cells, decreasing their viability by 69% and 46%, respectively, while the butanol, methanol, and ethanol extracts had no effect. Besides the water extract, no other FD crude extract had any effect on the viability of the D24 melanoma cells.

In contrast, all the FD crude extracts decreased the cell viability for the normal keratinocytes (HaCat). Except for the ethanol extract, which only decreased the HaCat cell viability by 24%, all the extracts reduced the viability by between 64% (water) and 75% (methanol).

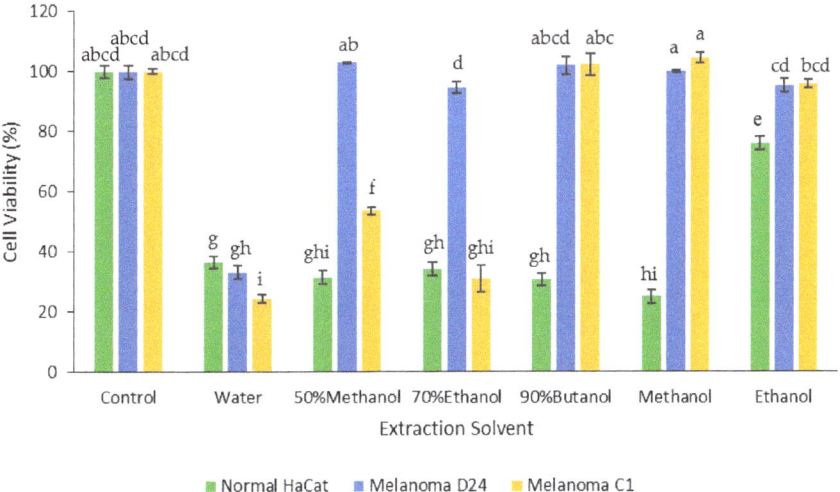

Figure 6. Effect of the FD crude extracts prepared with the different solvents on the cell viability of normal (HaCat) and melanoma (D24 and C1) cell lines after 48 h treatment. The values were the means ± SD of three replicate extractions for each solvent. Columns not sharing the same letter were significantly different at $p < 0.05$.

These results were consistent with the cellular changes observed using a phase contrast microscope. As seen in Figure 7, the control untreated HaCat keratinocytes were firmly attached with flattened oblong shapes (Figure 7A), the D24 melanoma cells were lightly attached with advanced elongations (Figure 7B), and the C1 melanoma cells were firmly attached and tightly packed with elongated processes (Figure 7C). In comparison to the untreated cells (Figure 7A–C), exposure of the cells to the various Gac seed extracts induced typical changes of cell death, such as cytoplasmic condensation, detached cells (red arrows in Figure 7), and cell disruption, to form apoptotic bodies (blue arrows in Figure 7).

The cellular changes observed with the water extract (Figure 7D–F) were consistent with the viability results (Figure 6) in that signs of morphological changes were seen for all three cell types. The 50% methanol and 70% ethanol extracts also caused substantial morphological changes to the C1 melanoma cells (Figure 7I,L) and HaCat cells (Figure 7G,J). The butanol and methanol extracts also caused substantial morphological changes to the HaCat cells (Figure 7M,P). In contrast, the ethanol extract had the least effect on the morphology of all three cells (Figure 7S–U) akin to controls.

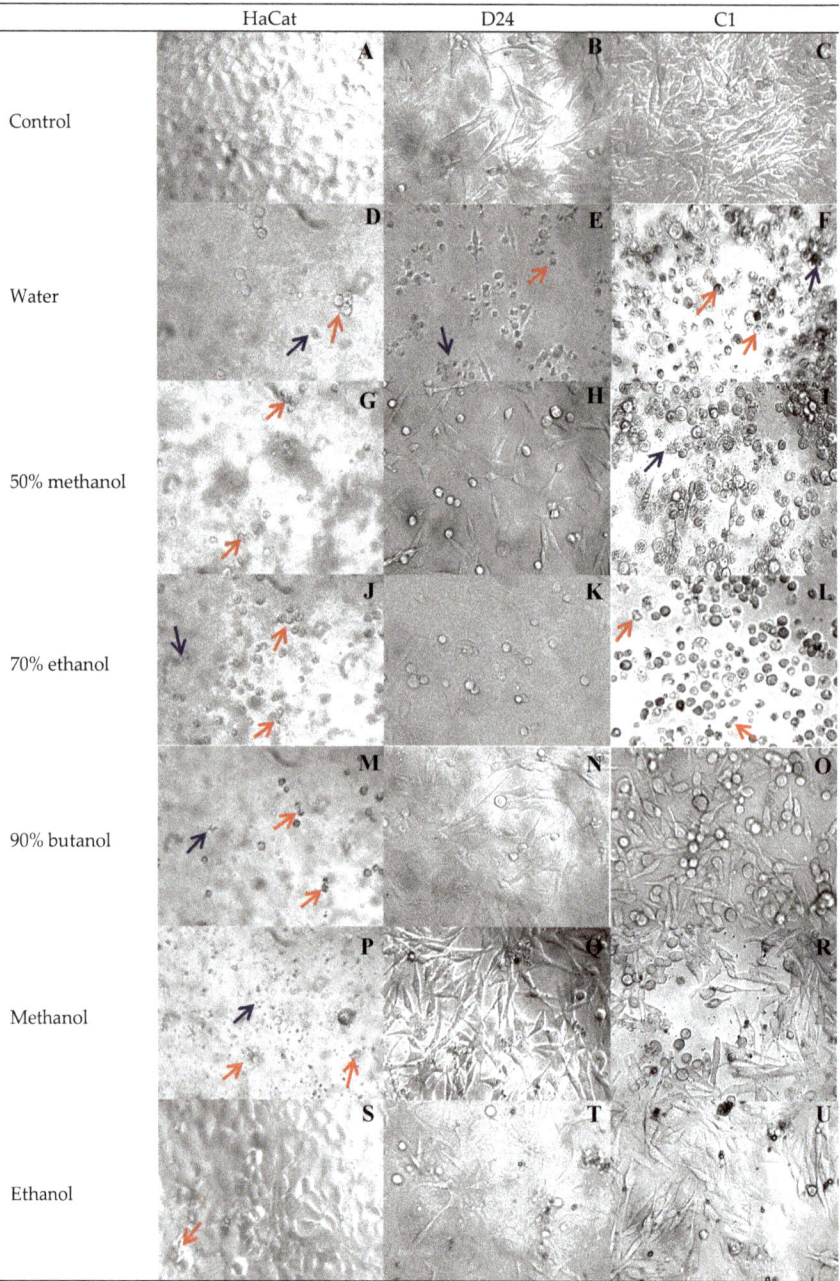

Figure 7. Morphological effects of different extraction solvents of Gac seed on HaCat (control) and melanoma D24 and C1 cell lines observed under a phase contrast microscope after 48 h treatment. Cytotoxicity is indicated by red arrows pointed to condensation and detached cells; blue arrows pointed to apoptotic bodies. Magnification: 100×.

The most sensitive cells were HaCat keratinocytes, while the least sensitive were the D24 melanoma cells, which had the least morphological changes when treated with all the solvent extracts, except for the water extract (Figure 7).

3.5. Correlations between Extract Yields, Bioactive Compounds, Antioxidant Activity, and Cancer Cell Viability across the FD Crude Extracts

TIA of the extracts was strongly and positively correlated with the extractable yield and the dry mass yield (Table 3, Figure 8). Essentially, the more material extracted, the higher the TIA, with the water extract having the highest values for both. TIA and extracted yields were also negatively correlated with the FRAP antioxidant activity and the viability of the C1 melanoma cells (Table 3, Figure 8). For example, almost 85% (r^2) of the variability in the C1 cell viability could be explained by variability in the TIA. In contrast, the C1 cell viability was positively correlated with the FRAP antioxidant activity. Therefore, the negative effect of the water extract on the C1 cell viability may be related to its high TIA but not FRAP activity.

Table 3. Coefficient of correlations (*r*) between yields, bioactive compounds, antioxidant activity, and cell viability across the Gac seed crude extracts.

	Yield		Bioactive Compound			Antioxidant Activity			Cell Viability		
	EY	DMY	TIA	TSC	TPC	ABTS	DPPH	FRAP	HaCat	D24	C1
EY	1.00										
DMY	0.98 [†]	1.00									
TIA	0.96 [‡]	0.97 [‡]	1.00								
TSC	−0.42	−0.50	−0.61	1.00							
TPC	0.51	0.49	0.31	0.36	1.00						
ABTS	0.48	0.43	0.29	0.44	0.97 [†]	1.00					
DPPH	−0.52	−0.58	−0.66	0.81 [§]	0.37	0.46	1.00				
FRAP	−0.93 [‡]	−0.89 [§]	−0.88 [§]	0.19	−0.48	−0.50	0.44	1.00			
HaCat	−0.42	−0.35	−0.22	−0.63	−0.73	−0.78	−0.28	0.63	1.00		
D24	−0.79	−0.80	−0.77	0.65	−0.28	−0.13	0.69	0.56	−0.01	1.00	
C1	−0.88 [§]	−0.83 [§]	−0.92 [§]	0.53	−0.23	−0.26	0.50	0.83 [§]	0.18	0.61	1.00

[†] $p < 0.001$, [‡] $p < 0.01$, [§] $p < 0.05$, EY: Extraction yield; DMY: Dry mass yield; TIA: Trypsin inhibitor activity; TSC: Total saponin content; TPC: Total phenolic content; ABTS: 2,2′-Azino-bis(3-ethylbenzothiazoline-6-sulfonic acid) assay; DPPH: 2,2-diphenyl-1-picrylhydrazyl assay; FRAP: ferric reducing antioxidant power assay.

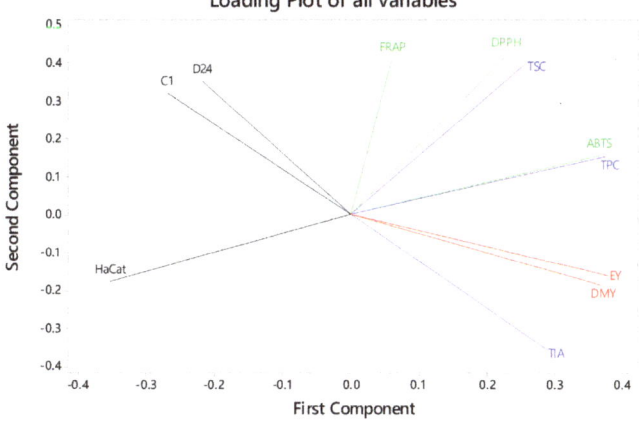

Figure 8. Correlations between extraction yields (red lines), bioactive compounds (blue lines), antioxidant activity (green lines), and cell viability (black lines) from Gac seed crude extracts.

There were positive correlations between the TSC with DPPH antioxidant activity, and TPC with ABTS antioxidant activity (Table 3, Figure 8). However, there were no significant correlations between these bioactive compounds and any other variables, including the effects of the extracts on cytotoxicity for both C1 and D24 cancer cells (Table 3, Figure 8). Furthermore, there were no other significant correlations between any of the other measured parameters.

4. Discussion

Gac seeds have long been used in traditional medicine as a remedy for numerous conditions. Several bioactive constituents have been identified in Gac seeds, such as trypsin inhibitors, saponins, and phenolics. In this study, the extraction of these bioactive constituents with different solvents was investigated and their relationships with antioxidant activity and anticancer potential were explored. The results revealed that the water extract had the highest anticancer potential, which may be related to its high content of trypsin inhibitors but not to its antioxidant activity.

The water extract from defatted Gac seeds had the highest anticancer potential, reducing the growth of the melanoma cells compared to the control. This is consistent with the finding that a water extract from Gac seeds was the best extract for supressing the migration and invasion of a breast cancer cell line [18]. Water extracts from Gac aril have also been shown to suppress the viability of colon, liver [17], and melanoma [41] cancer cell lines. Compared to the previous study [17], where the Gac aril water extract at 1.24 mg/mL inhibited colon and liver cancer cells by 38 and 45%, respectively, in the present study, the water extract at the much lower concentration of 0.2 mg/mL had a significantly higher anticancer activity of 67% and 75% for the D24 and C1 melanoma cells, respectively. This suggests that water is not only safe and inexpensive, but it is also a highly efficient solvent for extracting compounds with anticancer potential from Gac, especially Gac seeds. The use of water as the extraction solvent also means that the methodology is widely accessible to more people, particularly in rural and underdeveloped countries that do not have access to organic solvents and processing facilities.

The water extract also had the highest TIA value, which was likely due to the presence of trypsin inhibitor proteins because Gac seeds are known to contain trypsin inhibitor peptides that are soluble in buffered aqueous solvents [31,33,42]. The strong inverse correlation between TIA and the viability of the C1 melanoma cells also suggests that trypsin inhibitors were involved in the water extract's anticancer potential against these cells. The known Gac seed trypsin inhibitors have a low molecular weight of 3–4 kDa with a compact cyclic conformation [6,21], which can make it easy for them to penetrate into cancer cells and illicit cytotoxicity [43]. However, this is also consistent with the known anticancer potential of bigger proteins from Gac aril (35 kDa) [17] and other seeds, such as soybeans [44], which has been studied extensively [26,45–47].

However, although the water extract was the only extract to decrease the viability of the D24 melanoma cells, an inverse correlation between TIA and the viability of the D24 cells was not seen ($p = 0.07$) mainly because the 50% methanol and the 70% ethanol extracts had no activity against this cell line while they had activity against the C1 melanoma cell line. This could be due to the D24 cells, which have a mutated BRAF oncogene, being more resistant [48] to the presence of trypsin inhibitors, and therefore, they could only be killed when the trypsin inhibitors reach a high enough concentration, for example, in the water extract compared to the lower concentrations in the other extracts. However, it could also be that the D24 cells, and maybe also the C1 cells, were affected by other water soluble constituents of the Gac seeds, for example cyclotides which do not have trypsin inhibition activity [6]. For example, although many Gac seed trypsin inhibitors are cyclotides, MCoCC-1, a 3.3 kDa cyclotide unique to Gac seeds, which does not have trypsin inhibitor activity, has been shown to exhibit high cytotoxicity against the human melanoma MM96L cell line [6]; cell survival was decreased 43% in the presence of 2 µM MCoCC-1. The TIA is a measure of trypsin inhibitors, which may be cyclotides because they are found in Gac seeds [21], but other cyclotides are also present in Gac seeds that are purported to have anticancer potential [6,22]; however, these may not have antitrypsin activity and therefore would not be measured by the TIA.

The higher antioxidant activity of the butanol extract was likely due to its high content of saponin and phenolic compounds; this solvent had the highest TSC and TPC values among the extracts. There were strong positive correlations between saponins with DPPH antioxidant activity and phenolics with ABTS antioxidant activity, but neither saponins nor phenolic compounds were related to the FRAP antioxidant activity. Therefore, the extracted Gac seed saponins and phenolic compounds acted as antioxidants through the mechanism of scavenging the free radicals produced by DPPH and ABTS [39] rather than the reduction of oxidised intermediates in the FRAP chain reaction or through chelation [39]. A similar correlation was also reported by Chan et al. [49] for saponins and phenolic compounds extracted from defatted kenaf seeds. In that study, butanol was the most effective solvent for the extraction of saponins and phenolics. This solvent was non-polar enough to dissolve the saponin aglycones [50] and the phenolic rings [11], yet polar enough to also interact with the carbohydrate end of the saponin molecules and the carboxyl groups of gallic acid and p-hydroxybenzoic acid, which are reported to be present in Gac seeds [11]. Because butanol is classified by the FDA as a Class 3 solvent [51] with no known human hazards and approved for pharmaceutical applications, the use of it as an extraction solvent is regarded as less toxic and of low risk to human health.

Despite the high saponins, phenolics, and antioxidant activity of the butanol extract, it did not exhibit any anticancer potential against the two melanoma cell lines. This observation was not consistent with previous findings, which showed that one of the triterpenoid compounds found in Gac seed oil, karounidiol [20], had anticancer potential [19] and tumor inhibition effects [52]. This compound, likely a saponin, may not have been at a high enough concentration in the present extracts because the Gac seed kernels were defatted before they were extracted with the various solvents, which was consistent with a study by Le et al. [53], who found that Gac seed saponins were mainly associated with the fat component of the seeds.

5. Conclusions

Gac seeds, which are mostly considered as a waste product, could be a potentially useful source of anticancer candidates due to their cytotoxic activity against specific melanoma cells. The utilisation of Gac seeds to produce an anticancer product could reduce the waste burden on the environment and add value to the Gac fruit, which is cultivated in an increasing number of countries. This study found that water is suitable for the recovery of trypsin inhibitors and the preparation of an extract with significant anticancer potential. Butanol was found to be suitable to produce an extract enriched in saponins and phenolic compounds and with a high antioxidant activity. However, further studies are needed to fully understand what specific compounds are involved in the bioactivity of Gac seeds and their mechanism of action in order to better define their potential applications in the nutraceutical and pharmaceutical industries.

Author Contributions: Conceptualization, A.V.L., M.H.N., and P.D.R.; Methodology, A.V.L. and T.T.H.; Validation, A.V.L. and T.T.H.; Formal analysis, A.V.L., T.T.H.; Investigation, A.V.L.; Data curation, A.V.L., T.T.H., and P.D.R.; Writing—original draft preparation, A.V.L.; Writing—review & editing, A.V.L., T.T.H., P.D.R., M.H.N., and S.E.P.; Supervision, P.D.R. and M.H.N.

Funding: This research received no external funding.

Acknowledgments: A.V.L. acknowledges the University of Newcastle and the Vietnamese Ministry of Education and Training (MOET) for their financial support.

Conflicts of Interest: The authors declare no conflict of interest.

References

1. Wimalasiri, D.; Piva, T.; Urban, S.; Huynh, T. Morphological and genetic diversity of *Momordica cochinchinensis* (Cucurbitaceae) in Vietnam and Thailand. *Genet. Resour. Crop Evol.* **2016**, *63*, 19–33. [CrossRef]
2. Behera, T.; John, K.J.; Bharathi, L.; Karuppaiyan, R. Momordica. In *Wild Crop Relatives: Genomic and Breeding Resources*; Kole, C., Ed.; Springer: Heidelberg, Germany; New York, NY, USA, 2011; pp. 217–246.
3. Chuyen, H.V.; Nguyen, M.H.; Roach, P.D.; Golding, J.B.; Parks, S.E. Gac fruit (*Momordica cochinchinensis* Spreng): A rich source of bioactive compounds and its potential health benefits. *Int. J. Food Sci. Technol.* **2015**, *50*, 567–577. [CrossRef]
4. Huynh, T.; Nguyen, M.H.; Dao, N. Biomedical importance of *Momordica cochinchinensis* (GAC) fruit and future applications. *BJSTR* **2018**, *8*. in press.
5. Masayo, I.; Hikaru, O.; Tatsuo, Y.; Masako, T.; Yoshie, R.; Shuji, H.; Kunihide, M.; Ryuichi, H. Studies on the constituents of *Momordica cochinchinensis* Spreng. I. Isolation and characterization of the seed saponins, Momordica saponins I and II. *Chem. Pharm. Bull.* **1985**, *33*, 464–478. [CrossRef]
6. Chan, L.Y.; Wang, C.K.L.; Major, J.M.; Greenwood, K.P.; Lewis, R.J.; Craik, D.J.; Daly, N.L. Isolation and characterization of peptides from *Momordica cochinchinensis* seeds. *J. Nat. Prod.* **2009**, *72*, 1453–1458. [CrossRef] [PubMed]
7. Wong, R.C.; Fong, W.; Ng, T. Multiple trypsin inhibitors from *Momordica cochinchinensis* seeds, the Chinese drug mubiezhi. *Peptides* **2004**, *25*, 163–169. [CrossRef] [PubMed]
8. Chan, L.Y.; He, W.; Tan, N.; Zeng, G.; Craik, D.J.; Daly, N.L. A new family of cystine knot peptides from the seeds of *Momordica cochinchinensis*. *Peptides* **2013**, *39*, 29–35. [CrossRef] [PubMed]
9. Gao, X.M. (Ed.) Mu Bie Zi (*Semen momordicae*). In *Chinese Materia Medica Beijing*; Traditional Chinese Materia Medica Press: Beijing, China, 2005; Volume 2, pp. 601–602.
10. Lin, Z.Y.; Liu, X.; Yang, F.; Yu, Y.Q. Structural characterization and identification of five triterpenoid saponins isolated from *Momordica cochinchinensis* extracts by liquid chromatography/tandem mass spectrometry. *Int. J. Mass Spectrom.* **2012**, *328*, 43–66. [CrossRef]
11. Kubola, J.; Siriamornpun, S. Phytochemicals and antioxidant activity of different fruit fractions (peel, pulp, aril and seed) of Thai gac (*Momordica cochinchinensis* Spreng). *Food Chem.* **2011**, *127*, 1138–1145. [CrossRef] [PubMed]
12. Kang, J.M.; Kim, N.; Kim, B.; Kim, J.-H.; Lee, B.-Y.; Park, J.H.; Lee, M.K.; Lee, H.S.; Jang, I.-J.; Kim, J.S.; et al. Gastroprotective action of cochinchina Momordica seed extract is mediated by activation of CGRP and inhibition of cPLA2/5-LOX pathway. *Dig. Dis. Sci.* **2009**, *54*, 2549–2560. [CrossRef] [PubMed]
13. Jung, K.; Chin, Y.-W.; Chung, Y.H.; Park, Y.H.; Yoo, H.; Min, D.S.; Lee, B.; Kim, J. Anti-gastritis and wound healing effects of Momordicae Semen extract and its active component. *Immunopharmacol. Immunotoxicol.* **2013**, *35*, 126–132. [CrossRef] [PubMed]
14. Kang, J.M.; Kim, N.; Kim, B.; Kim, J.-H.; Lee, B.-Y.; Park, J.H.; Lee, M.K.; Lee, H.S.; Kim, J.S.; Jung, H.C.; et al. Enhancement of gastric ulcer healing and angiogenesis by cochinchina Momordica seed extract in rats. *J. Korean Med. Sci.* **2010**, *25*, 875–881. [CrossRef] [PubMed]
15. Yu, J.S.; Kim, J.H.; Lee, S.; Jung, K.; Kim, K.H.; Cho, J.Y. Src/Syk-targeted anti-inflammatory actions of triterpenoidal saponins from Gac (*Momordica cochinchinensis*) Seeds. *Am. J. Chin. Med.* **2017**, 1–15. [CrossRef] [PubMed]
16. Jung, K.; Chin, Y.-W.; Yoon, K.D.; Chae, H.-S.; Kim, C.Y.; Yoo, H.; Kim, J. Anti-inflammatory properties of a triterpenoidal glycoside from Momordica cochinchinensis in LPS-stimulated macrophages. *Immunopharmacol. Immunotoxicol.* **2013**, *35*, 8–14. [CrossRef] [PubMed]
17. Tien, P.G.; Kayama, F.; Konishi, F.; Tamemoto, H.; Kasono, K.; Hung, N.T.; Kuroki, M.; Ishikawa, S.E.; Van Nguyen, C.; Kawakami, M. Inhibition of tumor growth and angiogenesis by water extract of Gac fruit (*Momordica cochinchinensis* Spreng). *Int. J. Oncol.* **2005**, *26*, 881–889. [CrossRef] [PubMed]
18. Zheng, L.; Zhang, Y.-M.; Zhan, Y.-Z.; Liu, C.-X. *Momordica cochinchinensis* seed extracts suppress migration and invasion of human breast cancer ZR-75-30 cells via down-regulating MMP-2 and MMP-9. *Asian Pac. J. Cancer Prev.* **2014**, *15*, 1105–1110. [CrossRef] [PubMed]
19. Akihisa, T.; Tokuda, H.; Ichiishi, E.; Mukainaka, T.; Toriumi, M.; Ukiya, M.; Yasukawa, K.; Nishino, H. Anti-tumor promoting effects of multiflorane-type triterpenoids and cytotoxic activity of karounidiol against human cancer cell lines. *Cancer Lett.* **2001**, *173*, 9–14. [CrossRef]

20. Kan, L.; Hu, Q.; Chao, Z.; Song, X.; Cao, X. Chemical constituents of unsaponifiable matter from seed oil of *Momordica cochinchinensis*. *China J. Chin. Mater. Med.* **2006**, *31*, 1441–1444.
21. Hernandez, J.F.; Gagnon, J.; Chiche, L.; Nguyen, T.M.; Andrieu, J.P.; Heitz, A.; Trinh Hong, T.; Pham, T.T.; Le Nguyen, D. Squash trypsin inhibitors from *Momordica cochinchinensis* exhibit an atypical macrocyclic structure. *Biochemistry* **2000**, *39*, 5722–5730. [CrossRef] [PubMed]
22. Weidmann, J.; Craik, D.J. Discovery, structure, function, and applications of cyclotides: Circular proteins from plants. *J. Exp. Bot.* **2016**, *67*, 4801–4812. [CrossRef] [PubMed]
23. Sever, N.; Filipic, M.; Brzin, J.; Lah, T.T. Effect of cysteine proteinase inhibitors on murine B16 melanoma cell invasion in vitro. *Biol. Chem.* **2002**, *383*, 839–842. [CrossRef] [PubMed]
24. Heidtmann, H.-H.; Salge, U.; Abrahamson, M.; Bencina, M.; Kastelic, L.; Kopitar-Jerala, N.; Turk, V.; Lah, T.T. Cathepsin B and cysteine proteinase inhibitors in human lung cancer cell lines. *Clin. Exp. Metastasis* **1997**, *15*, 368–381. [CrossRef] [PubMed]
25. Clawson, G.A. Protease inhibitors and carcinogenesis: A review. *Cancer Investig.* **1996**, *14*, 597–608. [CrossRef]
26. Hocman, G. Chemoprevention of cancer: Protease inhibitors. *Int. J. Biochem.* **1992**, *24*, 1365–1375. [CrossRef]
27. Shamsi, T.N.; Parveen, R.; Afreen, S.; Azam, M.; Sen, P.; Sharma, Y.; Haque, Q.M.R.; Fatma, T.; Manzoor, N.; Fatima, S. Trypsin inhibitors from *Cajanus cajan* and *Phaseolus limensis* possess antioxidant, anti-Inflammatory, and antibacterial activity. *J. Diet. Suppl.* **2018**, 1–12. [CrossRef] [PubMed]
28. Samuelsson, G.; Kyerematen, G.; Farah, M.H. Preliminary chemical characterization of pharmacologically active compounds in aqueous plant extracts. *J. Ethnopharmacol.* **1985**, *14*, 193–201. [CrossRef]
29. Sasidharan, S.; Chen, Y.; Saravanan, D.; Sundram, K.; Latha, L.Y. Extraction, isolation and characterization of bioactive compounds from plants' extracts. *Afr. J. Tradit. Complement. Altern. Med.* **2011**, *8*, 1–10. [CrossRef] [PubMed]
30. Cheok, C.Y.; Salman, H.A.K.; Sulaiman, R. Extraction and quantification of saponins: A review. *Food Res. Int.* **2014**, *59*, 16–40. [CrossRef]
31. Mahatmanto, T.; Poth, A.G.; Mylne, J.S.; Craik, D.J. A comparative study of extraction methods reveals preferred solvents for cystine knot peptide isolation from *Momordica cochinchinensis* seeds. *Fitoterapia* **2014**, *95*, 22–33. [CrossRef] [PubMed]
32. Abascal, K.; Ganora, L.; Yarnell, E. The effect of freeze-drying and its implications for botanical medicine: A review. *Phytother. Res.* **2005**, *19*, 655–660. [CrossRef] [PubMed]
33. Klomklao, S.; Benjakul, S.; Kishimura, H.; Chaijan, M. Extraction, purification and properties of trypsin inhibitor from Thai mung bean (*Vigna radiata* (L.) R. Wilczek). *Food Chem.* **2011**, *129*, 1348–1354. [CrossRef]
34. Le, A.V.; Parks, S.E.; Nguyen, M.H.; Roach, P.D. Effect of solvents and extraction methods on recovery of bioactive compounds from defatted Gac (*Momordica cochinchinensis* Spreng.) seeds. *Separations* **2018**, *5*, 39. [CrossRef]
35. Makkar, H.P.; Siddhuraju, P.; Becker, K. Trypsin Inhibitor. In *Plant Secondary Metabolites*; Humana Press: New York, NY, USA, 2007; pp. 1–6.
36. Stauffer, C.E. Measuring trypsin inhibitor in soy meal: Suggested improvements in the standard method. *Cereal Chem.* **1990**, *67*, 296–302.
37. Tan, S.P.; Tuyen, K.C.; Parks, S.E.; Stathopoulos, C.E.; Roach, P.D. Effects of the spray-drying temperatures on the physiochemical properties of an encapsulated bitter melon aqueous extract powder. *Powder Technol.* **2015**, *281*, 65–75. [CrossRef]
38. Tan, S.P.; Vuong, Q.V.; Stathopoulos, C.E.; Parks, S.E.; Roach, P.D. Optimized aqueous extraction of saponins from bitter melon for production of a saponin-enriched bitter melon powder. *J. Food Sci.* **2014**, *79*, E1372–E1381. [CrossRef] [PubMed]
39. Thaipong, K.; Boonprakob, U.; Crosby, K.; Cisneros-Zevallos, L.; Byrne, D.H. Comparison of ABTS, DPPH, FRAP, and ORAC assays for estimating antioxidant activity from guava fruit extracts. *J. Food Compost. Anal.* **2006**, *19*, 669–675. [CrossRef]
40. Ishiyama, M.; Tominaga, H.; Shiga, M.; Sasamoto, K.; Ohkura, Y.; Ueno, K. A combined assay of cell vability and in vitro cytotoxicity with a highly water-soluble tetrazolium salt, neutral red and crystal violet. *Biol. Pharm Bull.* **1996**, *19*, 1518–1520. [CrossRef] [PubMed]
41. Wimalasiri, D. Genetic Diversity, Nutritional and Biological Activity of *Momordica cochinchinensis* (Cucurbitaceae). Ph.D. Thesis, RMIT University, Melbourne, Australia, 2015.

42. Arimatsu, P.; Sawangsook, O. Purification and characterization of Trypsin inhibitor from *Momordica cochinchinensis* Spreng. seed and its effects to Spodoptera litura. *Asian J. Plant Sci.* **2012**, *11*, 195–199. [CrossRef]
43. Cascales, L.; Henriques, S.T.; Kerr, M.C.; Huang, Y.-H.; Sweet, M.J.; Daly, N.L.; Craik, D.J. Identification and characterization of a new family of cell-penetrating peptides cyclic cell-penetrating peptides. *J. Biol. Chem.* **2011**, *286*, 36932–36943. [CrossRef] [PubMed]
44. Anderson, R.L.; Wolf, W.J. Compositional changes in trypsin inhibitors, phytic acid, saponins and isoflavones related to soybean processing. *J. Nutr.* **1995**, *125*, 581S. [CrossRef] [PubMed]
45. Birk, Y. *Plant Protease Inhibitors as Cancer Chemopreventive Agents*; Springer: Berlin, Germany, 2003; ISBN 978-3-642-05514-0.
46. Troll, W.; Kennedy, A.R. *Protease Inhibitors as Cancer Chemopreventive Agents*; Plenum Pub Corp: New York, NY, USA, 1993; ISBN 0306443902.
47. Kennedy, A.R. Chemopreventive agents: Protease inhibitors. *Pharmacol. Ther.* **1998**, *78*, 167–209. [CrossRef]
48. Housman, G.; Byler, S.; Heerboth, S.; Lapinska, K.; Longacre, M.; Snyder, N.; Sarkar, S. Drug resistance in cancer: An overview. *Cancers* **2014**, *6*, 1769–1792. [CrossRef] [PubMed]
49. Chan, K.W.; Iqbal, S.; Khong, N.M.; Ooi, D.-J.; Ismail, M. Antioxidant activity of phenolics–saponins rich fraction prepared from defatted kenaf seed meal. *LWT-Food Sci. Technol.* **2014**, *56*, 181–186. [CrossRef]
50. Hostettmann, K.; Marston, A. *Chemistry and Pharmacology of Natural Products, Saponin*; Cambridge University Press: Cambridge, NY, USA, 1995; ISBN 0-521-32970-1.
51. US Food and Drug Administration (FDA). *Guidance for Industry*; USHaH Services, Ed.; US Food and Drug Administration (FDA): Silver Spring, MD, USA, 2012.
52. Yasukawa, K.; Akihisa, T.; Tamura, T.; Takido, M. Inhibitory effect of karounidiol on 12-O-tetradecanoylphorbol-13-acetate-induced tumor promotion. *Biol. Pharm Bull.* **1994**, *17*, 460–462. [CrossRef] [PubMed]
53. Le, A.V.; Parks, S.E.; Nguyen, M.H.; Roach, P.D. Optimisation of the microwave-assisted ethanol extraction of saponins from Gac (*Momordica cochinchinensis* Spreng) seeds. *Medicines* **2018**, *5*, 70. [CrossRef] [PubMed]

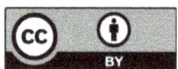

© 2018 by the authors. Licensee MDPI, Basel, Switzerland. This article is an open access article distributed under the terms and conditions of the Creative Commons Attribution (CC BY) license (http://creativecommons.org/licenses/by/4.0/).

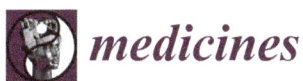

Review

Differential Methylation and Acetylation as the Epigenetic Basis of Resveratrol's Anticancer Activity

Mohd Farhan [1], Mohammad Fahad Ullah [2], Mohd Faisal [3], Ammad Ahmad Farooqi [4], Uteuliyev Yerzhan Sabitaliyevich [5], Bernhard Biersack [6] and Aamir Ahmad [7,*]

1. College of Basic Sciences, King Faisal University, Hofuf 400-Al Ahsa-31982, Saudi Arabia; mfarhan@kfu.edu.sa
2. Department of Medical Laboratory Technology, Faculty of Applied Medical Sciences, University of Tabuk, P.O. Box 741, Tabuk 71491, Saudi Arabia; m.ullah@ut.edu.sa
3. Department of Psychiatry, University Hospital Limerick, Limerick V94 T9PX, Ireland; mohd.faisal@hse.ie
4. Institute of Biomedical and Genetic Engineering (IBGE), Islamabad 44000, Pakistan; ammadfarooqi@rlmclahore.com
5. Department of Postgraduate Education and Research, Kazakhstan Medical University KSPH, Almaty 050004, Kazakhstan; e.uteuliyev@ksph.kz
6. Organic Chemistry Laboratory, Department of Chemistry, University of Bayreuth, Universitaetsstrasse 30, 95447 Bayreuth, Germany; bernhard.biersack@yahoo.com
7. Department of Oncologic Sciences, Mitchell Cancer Institute, University of South Alabama, Mobile, AL 36604, USA
* Correspondence: aahmad@health.southalabama.edu

Received: 11 January 2019; Accepted: 11 February 2019; Published: 13 February 2019

Abstract: Numerous studies support the potent anticancer activity of resveratrol and its regulation of key oncogenic signaling pathways. Additionally, the activation of sirtuin 1, a deacetylase, by resveratrol has been known for many years, making resveratrol perhaps one of the earliest nutraceuticals with associated epigenetic activity. Such epigenetic regulation by resveratrol, and the mechanism thereof, has attracted much attention in the past decade. Focusing on methylation and acetylation, the two classical epigenetic regulations, we showcase the potential of resveratrol as an effective anticancer agent by virtue of its ability to induce differential epigenetic changes. We discuss the de-repression of tumor suppressors such as BRCA-1, nuclear factor erythroid 2-related factor 2 (NRF2) and Ras Associated Domain family-1α (RASSF-1α) by methylation, PAX1 by acetylation and the phosphatase and tensin homologue (PTEN) by both methylation and acetylation, in addition to the epigenetic regulation of oncogenic NF-κB and STAT3 signaling by resveratrol. Further, we evaluate the literature supporting the potentiation of HDAC inhibitors and the inhibition of DNMTs by resveratrol in different human cancers. This discussion underlines a robust epigenetic activity of resveratrol that warrants further evaluation, particularly in clinical settings.

Keywords: resveratrol; epigenetic; methylation; acetylation

1. Introduction

Resveratrol (3,5,4'-trihydroxy-*trans*-stilbene) (Figure 1) is a naturally occurring polyphenol found in peanuts and the skin of grapes and berries. It is a phytoalexin produced in response to injury, ultraviolet radiation or a pathogen attack. The initial interest in resveratrol was because of its antioxidant properties [1], which led to the recognition of its chemopreventive ability [2]. Resveratrol was also found to generate reactive oxygen species, leading to effective anticancer activity through a prooxidant mechanism [3,4] which also happens to be a hallmark of several other polyphenols [5–7]. It is now believed that resveratrol exhibits both antioxidant and prooxidant properties [8–10], which depend largely on the tumor microenvironment and the presence of transition metal ions, particularly copper ions. Besides its anticancer properties, resveratrol has also been investigated to explain the 'French paradox' [11], a phenomenon of the relatively low incidence of coronary heart diseases in the French population despite a diet rich in saturated fats, perhaps due to the consumption of red wine with high resveratrol content.

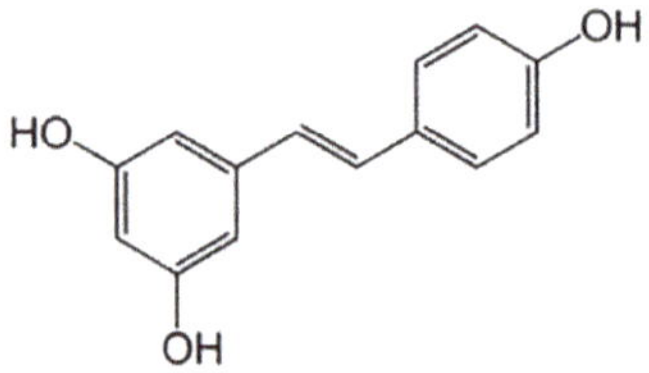

Figure 1. Chemical structure of resveratrol.

The realization of the potent anticancer properties of resveratrol was followed by numerous investigations into the various signaling pathways that it affects, leading to the observed effects [12–17]. In recent years, the focus of cancer research has shifted to stem cells, epithelial-to-mesenchymal transition (EMT) and epigenetic regulation, even in the context of lead compounds such as resveratrol that have a natural origin. Accordingly, a number of studies have documented the ability of resveratrol to affect stem cell populations [18,19] and EMT [20,21]. This article focuses on epigenetic regulation by resveratrol, which is increasingly being proposed as contributing to its anticancer properties.

2. Epigenetic Regulation by Resveratrol

Even though 'epigenetics' was originally intended to define heritable changes in phenotypes that were independent of changes in the DNA sequence, the meaning of this word has now considerably broadened to describe the alterations in human chromatin that influence DNA-templated processes [22,23]. Epigenetic changes do not result in any changes in the DNA sequence, but can still have lasting effects on gene expression. Epigenetic changes involve at least four known modifications of DNA and sixteen classes of histone modifications [22–24].

A number of studies have recognized the effects of nutraceuticals, including polyphenol resveratrol, on the epigenetic machinery in humans [25–35]. Resveratrol can modulate epigenetic patterns by altering the levels of S-adenosylmethionine and S-adenosylhomocysteine or by directing the enzymes that catalyze DNA methylation and histone modifications [27]. It also activates the deacetylase sirtuin and regulates oncogenic and tumor suppressor micro-RNAs [36]. Methylation and acetylation are two classical epigenetic modifications, and these will be the subject of our discussion in this article as we showcase the epigenetic basis of the anticancer action of resveratrol.

3. Methylation

The DNA methylation of gene promoters has a profound effect on their eventual expression and function. Differential DNA methylation can lead to a disease condition in healthy phenotypes. This is particularly true for cancer wherein the differential DNA methylation of the promoters of oncogenes and tumor suppressor genes helps maintain a delicate balance. The increased (hyper) methylation of promoter CpG islands causes gene silencing, while the decreased (hypo) methylation of promoter CpG islands leads to the expression of the gene.

3.1. Breast Cancer

Breast cancer is a widely studied cancer when it comes to epigenetic regulation, particularly differential methylation, by resveratrol. Studies have been conducted to elucidate the genome-wide methylation patterns after resveratrol treatment, and there have also been efforts to understand the epigenetic basis of the de-repression of tumor suppressors by resveratrol. The subsection to follow will focus on this activity of resveratrol.

3.1.1. Genome-Wide Analyses

A study on the genome-wide methylation-modifying effects of resveratrol, which involved exposing MCF10CA1h and MCF10CA1a cells to resveratrol for 9 days followed by Illumina 450K array analysis, revealed a profound effect of resveratrol on genome-wide DNA methylation with approximately 75% differentially methylated genes being hypermethylated [37]. This study evaluated the epigenetic activity of not only resveratrol but also pterostilbene, an analog of resveratrol. While treatment with resveratrol was done at a dose of 15 µM, pterostilbene treatment was at a 7 µM dose. The compounds targeted genes that are over-expressed in tumors because of DNA hypomethylation. Since increased DNA methylation results in the silencing of genes, it makes sense that the resveratrol-induced hypermethylated genes have predominantly oncogenic functions [37], such as the Notch signaling pathway. However, in another study that also looked at genome-wide DNA methylation after resveratrol treatment (in this case, 24 h and 48 h treatment), only about 12.5% of CpG loci were found to be differentially methylated by resveratrol [38]. This study used MDA-MB-231 breast cancer cells and the concentration of resveratrol was 100 µM. Additionally, this study predominantly found DNA hypomethylation by resveratrol. It is possible that the differences in genome-wide DNA methylation (75% vs. 12.5%) in these two studies might be reflective of the different experimental setups, in particular, the time-durations of the resveratrol treatment as well as the doses used, with longer treatment leading to substantially more methylation.

3.1.2. Effects on Tumor Suppressors

Tumor suppressor genes are typically inactivated at the onset of tumorigenesis and, therefore, their reactivation by anticancer therapy is a mechanism through which tumor progression can be controlled. Several studies have documented the epigenetic reactivation of the tumor suppressor genes by resveratrol in breast cancer (Figure 2), as discussed below.

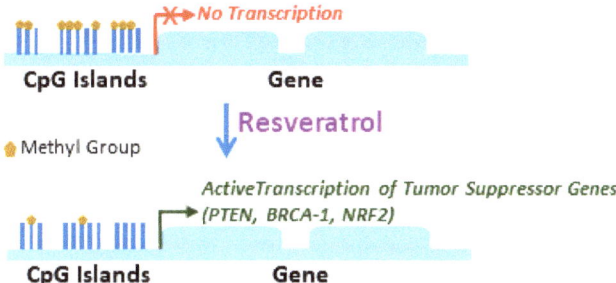

Figure 2. Activation of tumor suppressor genes by resveratrol through promoter DNA hypomethylation. The CpG islands in the DNA promoter regions of the tumor suppressor genes are hypermethylated resulting in their silencing. De-methylation of these CpG islands by resveratrol results in the activation of transcription and the eventual expression of tumor suppressor genes such as the phosphatase and tensin homologue (PTEN), BRCA-1 and nuclear factor erythroid 2-related factor 2 (NRF2).

Phosphatase and tensin homologue (PTEN) is a well-characterized tumor suppressor in breast cancer [39]. In one of the earlier studies describing an effect of resveratrol on promoter DNA methylation, it was reported that resveratrol was highly efficient in reducing PTEN promoter DNA methylation in MCF7 breast cancer cells [40]. Since reduced DNA methylation leads to gene expression, this action of resveratrol induced the expression of PTEN which could explain its anticancer effects. Further, it was reported that the epigenetic effects were complex as not only PTEN was induced but the cell cycle regulator p21 was up-regulated as well, in addition to the down-regulation of DNMT (DNA methyltransferase). This is interesting because DNA methyltransferases increase methylation. Thus, it appears that resveratrol is able to reduce DNA methylation possibly through two different ways—by reducing methylation and by inducing de-methylation.

BRCA-1 (breast cancer type 1) is another tumor suppressor gene. Its expression is known to be regulated by epigenetic mechanisms. In a study that demonstrated the effects of resveratrol on BRCA-1 methylation [41], it was shown that exposure of breast cancer cells MCF7 to tumor promoter TCDD (2,3,7,8 tetrachlorodibenzo-p-dioxin) resulted in the hypermethylation of BRCA-1 promoter CpG island concomitant with an increased association of trimethylated histone H3K9 and DNMTs, namely DNMT1, DNMT3a and DNMT3b, with BRCA-1 promoter. Resveratrol, at physiologically relevant doses, was able to repress these TCDD effects. In a follow-up study, the research group evaluated the effects of TCDD alone, and in combination with resveratrol, on pregnant Sprague–Dawley rats [42]. It was found that, similar to in vitro observations in MCF7 cells, gestational exposure to TCDD led to the reduced DNA CpG island methylation of BRCA-1 promoter in the mammary tissues of the offspring, which was preceded by the occupation of BRCA-1 promoter by DNMT-1. Also, confirming a possible therapeutic role, resveratrol was found to partially attenuate TCDD effects [42].

Nuclear factor erythroid 2-related factor 2 (NRF2) is also a tumor suppressor that is epigenetically regulated by resveratrol. In a study that looked at the effects of resveratrol on E2 (17β-estradiol)-induced carcinogenesis [43], resveratrol alone up-regulated NRF2 in mammary tissues of rats, and attenuated the repressive effects of E2 on NRF2. E2 suppressed NRF2 through DNA methylation, an activity that was inhibited by resveratrol, thus providing further evidence in support of its regulation of promoter DNA methylation in breast cancer.

3.1.3. DNMTs as Mediators of Resveratrol Effects in Breast Cancer

There is much evidence supporting an inhibitory effect of resveratrol against DNMTs [40,41,44–46]. However, most of the evidence comes from in vitro studies. To validate these findings, a pilot study was conducted that enrolled 39 women with increased breast cancer risk [47]. The subjects were divided into three groups—placebo and those receiving 5 or 50 mg resveratrol. Resveratrol was administered twice daily for twelve weeks and the focus was on the DNA methylation of four cancer-related genes—p16, Ras Associated Domain family-1α (RASSF-1α), Adenomatous Polyposis Coli (APC) and Cyclin D2 (CCND2). An inverse relationship between serum resveratrol levels and RASSF-1α methylation was observed, i.e., when resveratrol levels increased, the methylation of RASSF-1α decreased, thus leading to the expression of this tumor suppressor gene. In another study by this group [48], an in vivo effect of resveratrol on DNMT expression was examined in normal vs. tumor tissues. The model evaluated was ACI rats, an inbred line derived from the August and Copenhagen strains. An interesting observation was that resveratrol affected DNMT3b, but not DNMT1. Two different doses of resveratrol were tested and while DNMT3b differed in normal vs. tumor tissues of rats treated with low resveratrol, a high resveratrol dose resulted in decreased DNMT3b in tumor tissues with increased DNMT3b in the normal tissues [48]. This observation is a little different from the one performed in vitro in immortalized breast cancer epithelial cells, MCF10A [49], where resveratrol, at a non-cytotoxic dose, only induced subtle changes in the DNA methylation of eight pre-determined genes. However, the involvement of DNMT3b in resveratrol activity was also identified in a genome-wide DNA methylation study in breast cancer cells [37].

Further confirming the importance of targeting DNMTs in breast cancer patients, the elevated expression of DNMT transcripts was reported in a study that evaluated breast cancer tissues from 40 breast cancer patients and compared those with tissues from 10 paired normal breast tissues [50]. This study further confirmed the down-regulation of DNMT transcripts in vitro in breast cancer cells.

3.2. Glioma

Glioblastoma multiforme was the other malignancy where evidence of the effect of resveratrol on methylation was initially presented. It was shown that resveratrol could sensitize resistant glioblastoma T98G cells to temozolomide, inhibiting temozolomide IC-50 with increased apoptosis [51]. Interestingly, temozolomide-resistant cells have increased MGMT (O(6)-methylguanine-DNA-methyltransferase) activity and the protein expression of MGMT is an important determinant of temozolomide-resistance [51]. These results are suggestive of yet another DNA methylation-suppressing activity of resveratrol. In a recent report, inhibition of Wnt signaling has been identified as the mechanism by which resveratrol induces cell death in T98G cells [52]. Epigenetic regulation has been identified as one of the bases of perturbed Wnt signaling [53] and it is plausible that Wnt signaling might be another piece in the puzzle.

3.3. Lung Cancer

Lung cancer, the majority of which is non-small cell lung cancer (NSCLC), is the leading cause of cancer-related deaths in the United States, as well as worldwide. A number of studies have described the inhibitory effects of resveratrol against various lung cancer models [54–56], albeit, a majority of the studies have focused on NSCLC with little information on the other lung cancer types. In recent years, efforts have been made towards the personalized management of lung cancer [57], with a focus on epigenetics in such personalized therapy [58]. Further, it has recently been demonstrated that resveratrol can epigenetically regulate the expression of zinc finger protein36 (ZFP36) through differential DNA methylation [59]. Specifically, resveratrol reduced the methylation of ZFP36, resulting in its up-regulation in A549 NSCLC cells. A role of ZFP36 in human malignancies is increasingly being realized, making it an attractive target for therapy [60]. Thus, its epigenetic targeting by resveratrol further underlines the anticancer potential of resveratrol, particularly in lung cancer.

4. Acetylation

Even before the realization of the methylation potential of resveratrol, it has been known to modulate acetylation within the cellular microenvironment. A quarter century back, resveratrol was reported to be an activator of sirtuin-1 (SIRT1), the NAD-dependent deacetylase, marking its influence on acetylation, and thereby epigenetic regulation [61]. While the activity of resveratrol against Class III HDACs sirtuins is well characterized, it has been suggested that perhaps resveratrol possesses a pan-HDAC inhibitory property and can inhibit HDACs representing class I, class II as well as class IV [62]. Recently, resveratrol has been identified as an inhibitor of bromodomains [63] and the bromodomain and extraterminal (BET) family [64]. Bromodomains affect epigenetic machinery by recognizing lysine acetylation on histones, thereby functioning as epigenetic readers. The interactions of resveratrol with bromodomains open yet another mechanism of epigenetic regulation by resveratrol which is not yet fully explored. The next few subsections discuss the reported effects of resveratrol on the acetylation of different genes in various human cancers.

4.1. Breast Cancer

Acetylation and its impact on breast cancer progression is well appreciated. It is because of this knowledge that HDAC inhibitors still remain an attractive therapeutic strategy against breast cancers [65–67]. It is not only the HDAC inhibitors but also the inhibitors of HATs (histone acetyltransferases) that are being evaluated [68], which provides a good example of how dynamic the process of acetylation and deacetylation is, and how an imbalance can lead to tumor onset and progression. In a study [69] that is indicative of an intricate connection between methylation and acetylation, the two classical epigenetic modifications, it was reported that lysine acetylation within the signal transducer and activator of transcription 3 (STAT3) can impact the interaction of DNMT1 with STAT3 and is accompanied by the demethylation and, thereby, the re-expression of tumor suppressor genes. This study used resveratrol as an acetylation inhibitor and the observations in triple negative breast cancer (TNBC) were further confirmed in melanoma. TNBCs are characterized by the absence of the estrogen receptor (ER) and progesterone receptor (PR), as well as human epidermal growth factor receptor 2 (HER2), and it has been reported that the absence of the *ERα* gene in tumor cells is often a result of methylation [70]. With the observation that STAT3 is acetylated and, therefore, highly expressed in TNBCs, it was evaluated whether inhibiting STAT3 acetylation could reactivate ERα [69]. The TNBC cell line MDA-MB-468 was used as the model and it was observed that treatment with resveratrol significantly reduced STAT3 acetylation as well as ERα gene promoter DNA methylation (Figure 3). This resulted in the increased expression of ERα and the sensitization of otherwise resistant cells to the ER-targeted therapy, tamoxifen. Further, growth of in vivo tumors in mice was not significantly reduced by tamoxifen alone, as expected, but by the combinational treatment comprising resveratrol and tamoxifen, thus validating the in vitro findings [69]. As further evidence of the effect of resveratrol on acetylation in breast cancer, in MCF-7 breast cancer cells, resveratrol has been shown to induce H3 acetylation [71]. Thus, there seems to be evidence suggesting a modulatory effect of resveratrol on protein as well as histone acetylation.

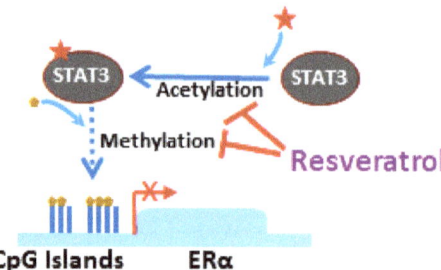

Figure 3. Epigenetic regulation in triple negative breast cancers (TNBCs). TNBCs are characterized by activated STAT3 signaling, involving acetylated STAT3. ERα signaling in TNBCs is silenced through promoter DNA hypermethylation which might be related to STAT3 acetylation but the mechanisms remain unclear (and are therefore shown with a dotted line). Resveratrol is an effective inhibitor of STAT3 acetylation as well as ERα promoter DNA methylation. Restoration of ER-signaling makes TNBC cells sensitive to the ER-targeting therapy, tamoxifen.

4.2. Cervical Cancer

In cervical cancer models, paired box gene1 (PAX1) is a tumor suppressor whose expression is repressed during tumorigenesis by DNA hypermethylation. In a study that evaluated the effect of nutraceuticals, including resveratrol, on the inhibition of cervical cancer through the reactivation of PAX1, it was reported that resveratrol was capable of reactivating PAX1 expression in Caski cells [72]. However, surprisingly, the reactivation of PAX1 was not found to be due to the effect of resveratrol on the DNA methylation of PAX1 promoter. Rather, it possibly involved the acetylation modulating ability of resveratrol through its regulation of HDAC activity. Similar to an effect of resveratrol on histone H3 acetylation in breast cancer cells above, resveratrol has been reported to induce H3 acetylation in HeLa cervical cancer cells as well [71]. Such an effect of resveratrol on H3 acetylation assumes significance given the proposed role of histone H3 acetylation as a prognostic marker for cervical cancer patients [73].

4.3. Colon Cancer

NF-κB signaling is known to be important to the progression of colon cancer [74], especially in resistance to cisplatin [75]. An increase in the protein acetylation of the NF-κB p65 subunit leads to the activation of the NF-κB pathway and its nuclear accumulation. Therefore, the inhibition of the acetylation of p65 can potentially be an effective strategy to check the growth of colon cancer as well as to overcome resistance to cisplatin. In an in vitro study performed in HK2 cells, resveratrol was found to decrease the protein acetylation of the p65 subunit, thus reversing the cell viability-inducing activity of cisplatin [76]. Such down-regulation of NF-κB protein acetylation by resveratrol in colorectal cells was confirmed in another study [77] and this resulted in reduced tumor invasion and metastasis because of the down regulation of NF-κB-regulated factors, such as MMP-9 and CXCR4.

4.4. Leukemia and Lymphoma

In leukemia, resveratrol can potentiate the activity of HDAC inhibitors [78], while in a Hodgkin lymphoma represented by L-428 cells, resveratrol can effectively induce apoptosis as well as cell cycle arrest [79]. As the mechanism, it was observed that resveratrol induced the tumor suppressor p53 through an increase in the p53 K373-acetylation (Table 1). Additionally, resveratrol treatment was found to induce the lysine acetylation of FOXO3a [79]. In leukemia U937 cells, resveratrol potentiates reactive oxygen species production by retinoic acid, particularly the production of superoxide anions, primarily through the up-regulation of the gp91-phox gene that is part of the membrane-bound cytochrome b_{558} [80]. As a mechanism, it was elucidated that resveratrol promoted acetylation within the promoter region of the gp91-phox gene, particularly the Lys-9 residues and Lys-14 residues of histone H3 within the chromatin surrounding the gene promoter.

Table 1. Epigenetic effects of resveratrol on tumor suppressors: mechanisms of their re-activation.

Tumor Suppressor	Cancer Type	Effect of Resveratrol	Reference
BRCA-1	Breast	Reduced promotor DNA methylation in vitro	[36]
		Reduced promotor DNA methylation in vivo	[37]
NRF2	Breast	Reduced promotor DNA methylation	[38]
p53	Lymphoma	Induced acetylation	[73]
	Prostate		[75]
PAX1	Cervical	Regulation of histone acetylation	[66]
PTEN	Breast	Reduced promoter DNA methylation	[35]
	Prostate	Acetylation and activation	[77]
RASSF-1α	Breast	Reduced DNA methylation	[42]

4.5. Prostate Cancer

In prostate cancer, metastasis-associated protein 1 (MTA1) is oncogenic with its expression correlating with tumor progression. It is itself involved in the transcriptional repression of target genes through the post-translational modifications of histones as well as non-histones by virtue of it being a part of the nucleosome remodeling deacetylation corepressor complex, the 'NuRD complex'. Resveratrol was shown to down-regulate MTA1, leading to acetylation and the activation of the tumor suppressor p53 through the destabilization of the corepressor complex [81]. The NuRD complex plays a role in maintaining chromatin conformation, which it achieves through the deacetylation of histone proteins [82]. HDAC1 and HDA2 are components of the NuRD complex, with the MTA1-HDAC1 subunit responsible for the deacetylation of histones by NuRD. With a direct regulation of MTA1, and the observation that HDAC1 was decreased in resveratrol-treated MTA1 immunoprecipitates, it is evident that resveratrol has a profound effect on histone acetylation. Further, the effects of resveratrol were similar to those of the HDAC inhibitor SAHA, thus underlying the acetylation-affecting epigenetic activity of resveratrol. The results were further confirmed in vivo in a follow-up study [83], and it was shown that the MTA1-mediated tumor progression was, in part, due to PTEN inactivation and that resveratrol could acetylate and reactivate PTEN [84] (Table 1).

Signaling through the androgen receptor (AR) is important in prostate cancer, even in the advanced castrate-resistant prostate cancers. In a study that specifically looked at the regulation of AR signaling by resveratrol, it was observed that treatment with 10 µM resveratrol for just 3 h inhibited the acetylation of AR and affected the binding of AR to the enhancer region of prostate-specific antigen (PSA) [85]. At a slightly longer treatment of 24 h, resveratrol inhibited the nuclear accumulation of AR as well. Given the important role that AR plays in prostate cancer, such epigenetic regulation of its activity and the effect on down-stream signaling by resveratrol is an encouraging finding that gives hope for its possible use as a therapy against prostate cancer.

5. Conclusions and Perspectives

While various cellular signaling pathways and genes (oncogenes as well as tumor suppressor genes) are still being evaluated as therapeutic targets of anticancer agents such as resveratrol, in recent years, attention has also turned to epigenetic regulation. In fact, epigenetic regulation of classical signaling pathways is increasingly being realized. For example, two of the very well characterized signaling pathways, NF-κB and STAT3, are epigenetically regulated by resveratrol [69,76,77,86]. This represents a fundamental evolution in our understanding with regards to the intricate regulation of oncogenic pathways. Our discussion on the topic, as presented in this article, detailed many studies that provided evidence supporting the epigenetic activity of resveratrol. However, resveratrol does not regulate gene expression only through epigenetic mechanisms. For example, in a study in acute lymphoblastic leukemia [87] that looked at the possible effect of resveratrol on the methylation of MDR1 (multidrug resistance gene 1), no evidence of the differential DNA methylation of MDR1 promoter by resveratrol was found. While resveratrol had a visible suppressive effect on MDR1, there did not seem to be any epigenetic perspective. This is a perfect reminder that not all regulation of gene expression and function by resveratrol has an epigenetic basis. Additionally, regulation through microRNAs (miRNAs) is within the realm of epigenetic regulation, but we decided to cover just the classical epigenetic mechanisms with regards to methylation and acetylation so as to keep the discussion more focused. Finally, the bioavailability of resveratrol still remains a concern, but that should not deter us from fully elucidating its mechanism of action and its potential as a viable anticancer lead. Several groups are working hard on improving the bioavailability through novel approaches and once they achieve success, resveratrol should be ready for further evaluations in clinical settings as an anticancer agent with multifaceted epigenetic activity.

Funding: Mohd Farhan is thankful to the Deanship of Scientific Research, King Faisal University, for a research grant through the Nasher track (186105).

Conflicts of Interest: The authors declare no conflict of interest.

References

1. Miller, N.J.; Rice-Evans, C.A. Antioxidant activity of resveratrol in red wine. *Clin. Chem.* **1995**, *41*, 1789. [PubMed]
2. Jang, M.; Cai, L.; Udeani, G.O.; Slowing, K.V.; Thomas, C.F.; Beecher, C.W.; Fong, H.H.; Farnsworth, N.R.; Kinghorn, A.D.; Mehta, R.G.; et al. Cancer chemopreventive activity of resveratrol, a natural product derived from grapes. *Science* **1997**, *275*, 218–220. [CrossRef] [PubMed]
3. Ahmad, A.; Farhan Asad, S.; Singh, S.; Hadi, S.M. DNA breakage by resveratrol and cu(ii): Reaction mechanism and bacteriophage inactivation. *Cancer Lett.* **2000**, *154*, 29–37. [CrossRef]
4. Ahmad, A.; Syed, F.A.; Singh, S.; Hadi, S.M. Prooxidant activity of resveratrol in the presence of copper ions: Mutagenicity in plasmid DNA. *Toxicol. Lett.* **2005**, *159*, 1–12. [CrossRef]
5. Khan, H.Y.; Zubair, H.; Faisal, M.; Ullah, M.F.; Farhan, M.; Sarkar, F.H.; Ahmad, A.; Hadi, S.M. Plant polyphenol induced cell death in human cancer cells involves mobilization of intracellular copper ions and reactive oxygen species generation: A mechanism for cancer chemopreventive action. *Mol. Nutr. Food Res.* **2014**, *58*, 437–446. [CrossRef] [PubMed]
6. Khan, H.Y.; Zubair, H.; Ullah, M.F.; Ahmad, A.; Hadi, S.M. A prooxidant mechanism for the anticancer and chemopreventive properties of plant polyphenols. *Curr. Drug Targets* **2012**, *13*, 1738–1749. [CrossRef] [PubMed]
7. Farhan, M.; Oves, M.; Chibber, S.; Hadi, S.M.; Ahmad, A. Mobilization of nuclear copper by green tea polyphenol epicatechin-3-gallate and subsequent prooxidant breakage of cellular DNA: Implications for cancer chemotherapy. *Int. J. Mol. Sci.* **2016**, *18*, 34. [CrossRef] [PubMed]
8. de la Lastra, C.A.; Villegas, I. Resveratrol as an antioxidant and pro-oxidant agent: Mechanisms and clinical implications. *Biochem. Soc. Trans.* **2007**, *35*, 1156–1160. [CrossRef] [PubMed]

9. Casey, S.C.; Amedei, A.; Aquilano, K.; Azmi, A.S.; Benencia, F.; Bhakta, D.; Bilsland, A.E.; Boosani, C.S.; Chen, S.; Ciriolo, M.R.; et al. Cancer prevention and therapy through the modulation of the tumor microenvironment. *Semin. Cancer Biol.* **2015**, *35*, S199–S223. [CrossRef] [PubMed]
10. Chen, C.Y.; Kao, C.L.; Liu, C.M. The cancer prevention, anti-inflammatory and anti-oxidation of bioactive phytochemicals targeting the tlr4 signaling pathway. *Int. J. Mol. Sci.* **2018**, *19*, 2729. [CrossRef]
11. Kopp, P. Resveratrol, a phytoestrogen found in red wine. A possible explanation for the conundrum of the 'french paradox'? *Eur. J. Endocrinol.* **1998**, *138*, 619–620. [CrossRef] [PubMed]
12. Shukla, Y.; Singh, R. Resveratrol and cellular mechanisms of cancer prevention. *Ann. N. Y. Acad. Sci.* **2011**, *1215*, 1–8. [CrossRef] [PubMed]
13. Yang, X.; Li, X.; Ren, J. From french paradox to cancer treatment: Anti-cancer activities and mechanisms of resveratrol. *Anti-Cancer Agents Med. Chem.* **2014**, *14*, 806–825. [CrossRef]
14. McCalley, A.E.; Kaja, S.; Payne, A.J.; Koulen, P. Resveratrol and calcium signaling: Molecular mechanisms and clinical relevance. *Molecules* **2014**, *19*, 7327–7340. [CrossRef] [PubMed]
15. Farooqi, A.A.; Wu, S.J.; Chang, Y.T.; Tang, J.Y.; Li, K.T.; Ismail, M.; Liaw, C.C.; Li, R.N.; Chang, H.W. Activation and inhibition of atm by phytochemicals: Awakening and sleeping the guardian angel naturally. *Arch. Immunol. Ther. Exp.* **2015**, *63*, 357–366. [CrossRef] [PubMed]
16. de Oliveira, M.R.; Nabavi, S.F.; Manayi, A.; Daglia, M.; Hajheydari, Z.; Nabavi, S.M. Resveratrol and the mitochondria: From triggering the intrinsic apoptotic pathway to inducing mitochondrial biogenesis, a mechanistic view. *Biochimi. Biophys. Acta* **2016**, *1860*, 727–745. [CrossRef] [PubMed]
17. Zhang, L.; Wen, X.; Li, M.; Li, S.; Zhao, H. Targeting cancer stem cells and signaling pathways by resveratrol and pterostilbene. *BioFactors* **2018**, *44*, 61–68. [CrossRef]
18. Sarkar, F.H.; Li, Y.; Wang, Z.; Kong, D. The role of nutraceuticals in the regulation of wnt and hedgehog signaling in cancer. *Cancer Metast. Rev.* **2010**, *29*, 383–394. [CrossRef]
19. McCubrey, J.A.; Lertpiriyapong, K.; Steelman, L.S.; Abrams, S.L.; Yang, L.V.; Murata, R.M.; Rosalen, P.L.; Scalisi, A.; Neri, L.M.; Cocco, L.; et al. Effects of resveratrol, curcumin, berberine and other nutraceuticals on aging, cancer development, cancer stem cells and micrornas. *Aging* **2017**, *9*, 1477–1536. [CrossRef]
20. Karimi Dermani, F.; Saidijam, M.; Amini, R.; Mahdavinezhad, A.; Heydari, K.; Najafi, R. Resveratrol inhibits proliferation, invasion, and epithelial-mesenchymal transition by increasing mir-200c expression in hct-116 colorectal cancer cells. *J. Cell. Biochem.* **2017**, *118*, 1547–1555. [CrossRef]
21. Xu, J.; Liu, D.; Niu, H.; Zhu, G.; Xu, Y.; Ye, D.; Li, J.; Zhang, Q. Resveratrol reverses doxorubicin resistance by inhibiting epithelial-mesenchymal transition (emt) through modulating pten/akt signaling pathway in gastric cancer. *J. Exp. Clin. Cancer Res.* **2017**, *36*, 19. [CrossRef] [PubMed]
22. Dawson, M.A.; Kouzarides, T. Cancer epigenetics: From mechanism to therapy. *Cell* **2012**, *150*, 12–27. [CrossRef] [PubMed]
23. Ahmad, A.; Li, Y.; Bao, B.; Kong, D.; Sarkar, F.H. Epigenetic regulation of mirna-cancer stem cells nexus by nutraceuticals. *Mol. Nutr. Food Res.* **2014**, *58*, 79–86. [CrossRef] [PubMed]
24. Baylin, S.B.; Jones, P.A. A decade of exploring the cancer epigenome—biological and translational implications. *Nat. Rev. Cancer* **2011**, *11*, 726–734. [CrossRef] [PubMed]
25. Vanden Berghe, W. Epigenetic impact of dietary polyphenols in cancer chemoprevention: Lifelong remodeling of our epigenomes. *Pharmacol. Res.* **2012**, *65*, 565–576. [CrossRef] [PubMed]
26. Hardy, T.M.; Tollefsbol, T.O. Epigenetic diet: Impact on the epigenome and cancer. *Epigenomics* **2011**, *3*, 503–518. [CrossRef] [PubMed]
27. Park, L.K.; Friso, S.; Choi, S.W. Nutritional influences on epigenetics and age-related disease. *Proc. Nutr. Soc.* **2012**, *71*, 75–83. [CrossRef] [PubMed]
28. Gerhauser, C. Cancer chemoprevention and nutriepigenetics: State of the art and future challenges. *Top. Curr. Chem.* **2013**, *329*, 73–132. [PubMed]
29. Wang, Y.; Li, Y.; Liu, X.; Cho, W.C. Genetic and epigenetic studies for determining molecular targets of natural product anticancer agents. *Curr. Cancer Drug Targets* **2013**, *13*, 506–518. [CrossRef] [PubMed]
30. Vahid, F.; Zand, H.; Nosrat-Mirshekarlou, E.; Najafi, R.; Hekmatdoost, A. The role dietary of bioactive compounds on the regulation of histone acetylases and deacetylases: A review. *Gene* **2015**, *562*, 8–15. [CrossRef] [PubMed]
31. Gao, Y.; Tollefsbol, T.O. Impact of epigenetic dietary components on cancer through histone modifications. *Curr. Med. Chem.* **2015**, *22*, 2051–2064. [CrossRef] [PubMed]

32. Kala, R.; Tollefsbol, T.O. A novel combinatorial epigenetic therapy using resveratrol and pterostilbene for restoring estrogen receptor-alpha (eralpha) expression in eralpha-negative breast cancer cells. *PLoS ONE* **2016**, *11*, e0155057. [CrossRef] [PubMed]
33. Fernandes, G.F.S.; Silva, G.D.B.; Pavan, A.R.; Chiba, D.E.; Chin, C.M.; Dos Santos, J.L. Epigenetic regulatory mechanisms induced by resveratrol. *Nutrients* **2017**, *9*, 1201. [CrossRef] [PubMed]
34. Lee, P.S.; Chiou, Y.S.; Ho, C.T.; Pan, M.H. Chemoprevention by resveratrol and pterostilbene: Targeting on epigenetic regulation. *BioFactors* **2018**, *44*, 26–35. [CrossRef] [PubMed]
35. Singh, A.K.; Bishayee, A.; Pandey, A.K. Targeting histone deacetylases with natural and synthetic agents: An emerging anticancer strategy. *Nutrients* **2018**, *10*, 731. [CrossRef]
36. Stefanska, B.; Karlic, H.; Varga, F.; Fabianowska-Majewska, K.; Haslberger, A. Epigenetic mechanisms in anti-cancer actions of bioactive food components–the implications in cancer prevention. *Br. J. Pharmacol.* **2012**, *167*, 279–297.
37. Lubecka, K.; Kurzava, L.; Flower, K.; Buvala, H.; Zhang, H.; Teegarden, D.; Camarillo, I.; Suderman, M.; Kuang, S.; Andrisani, O.; et al. Stilbenoids remodel the DNA methylation patterns in breast cancer cells and inhibit oncogenic notch signaling through epigenetic regulation of maml2 transcriptional activity. *Carcinogenesis* **2016**, *37*, 656–668. [CrossRef]
38. Medina-Aguilar, R.; Perez-Plasencia, C.; Marchat, L.A.; Gariglio, P.; Garcia Mena, J.; Rodriguez Cuevas, S.; Ruiz-Garcia, E.; Astudillo-de la Vega, H.; Hernandez Juarez, J.; Flores-Perez, A.; et al. Methylation landscape of human breast cancer cells in response to dietary compound resveratrol. *PLoS ONE* **2016**, *11*, e0157866. [CrossRef]
39. Ramaiah, M.J.; Vaishnave, S. Bmi1 and pten are key determinants of breast cancer therapy: A plausible therapeutic target in breast cancer. *Gene* **2018**, *678*, 302–311.
40. Stefanska, B.; Salame, P.; Bednarek, A.; Fabianowska-Majewska, K. Comparative effects of retinoic acid, vitamin d and resveratrol alone and in combination with adenosine analogues on methylation and expression of phosphatase and tensin homologue tumour suppressor gene in breast cancer cells. *Br. J. Nutr.* **2012**, *107*, 781–790. [CrossRef]
41. Papoutsis, A.J.; Borg, J.L.; Selmin, O.I.; Romagnolo, D.F. Brca-1 promoter hypermethylation and silencing induced by the aromatic hydrocarbon receptor-ligand tcdd are prevented by resveratrol in mcf-7 cells. *J. Nutr. Biochem.* **2012**, *23*, 1324–1332. [CrossRef] [PubMed]
42. Papoutsis, A.J.; Selmin, O.I.; Borg, J.L.; Romagnolo, D.F. Gestational exposure to the ahr agonist 2,3,7,8-tetrachlorodibenzo-p-dioxin induces brca-1 promoter hypermethylation and reduces brca-1 expression in mammary tissue of rat offspring: Preventive effects of resveratrol. *Mol. Carcinog.* **2015**, *54*, 261–269. [CrossRef] [PubMed]
43. Singh, B.; Shoulson, R.; Chatterjee, A.; Ronghe, A.; Bhat, N.K.; Dim, D.C.; Bhat, H.K. Resveratrol inhibits estrogen-induced breast carcinogenesis through induction of nrf2-mediated protective pathways. *Carcinogenesis* **2014**, *35*, 1872–1880. [CrossRef] [PubMed]
44. Singh, V.; Sharma, P.; Capalash, N. DNA methyltransferase-1 inhibitors as epigenetic therapy for cancer. *Curr. Cancer Drug Targets* **2013**, *13*, 379–399. [CrossRef] [PubMed]
45. Kala, R.; Shah, H.N.; Martin, S.L.; Tollefsbol, T.O. Epigenetic-based combinatorial resveratrol and pterostilbene alters DNA damage response by affecting sirt1 and dnmt enzyme expression, including sirt1-dependent gamma-h2ax and telomerase regulation in triple-negative breast cancer. *BMC Cancer* **2015**, *15*, 672. [CrossRef] [PubMed]
46. Gao, Y.; Tollefsbol, T.O. Combinational proanthocyanidins and resveratrol synergistically inhibit human breast cancer cells and impact epigenetic(-)mediating machinery. *Int. J. Mol. Sci.* **2018**, *19*, 2204. [CrossRef] [PubMed]
47. Zhu, W.; Qin, W.; Zhang, K.; Rottinghaus, G.E.; Chen, Y.C.; Kliethermes, B.; Sauter, E.R. Trans-resveratrol alters mammary promoter hypermethylation in women at increased risk for breast cancer. *Nutr. Cancer* **2012**, *64*, 393–400. [CrossRef]
48. Qin, W.; Zhang, K.; Clarke, K.; Weiland, T.; Sauter, E.R. Methylation and mirna effects of resveratrol on mammary tumors vs. Normal tissue. *Nutr. Cancer* **2014**, *66*, 270–277. [CrossRef]
49. Beetch, M.; Lubecka, K.; Kristofzski, H.; Suderman, M.; Stefanska, B. Subtle alterations in DNA methylation patterns in normal cells in response to dietary stilbenoids. *Mol. Nutr. Food Res.* **2018**, *2018*, e1800193. [CrossRef]

50. Mirza, S.; Sharma, G.; Parshad, R.; Gupta, S.D.; Pandya, P.; Ralhan, R. Expression of DNA methyltransferases in breast cancer patients and to analyze the effect of natural compounds on DNA methyltransferases and associated proteins. *J. Breast Cancer* **2013**, *16*, 23–31. [CrossRef]
51. Huang, H.; Lin, H.; Zhang, X.; Li, J. Resveratrol reverses temozolomide resistance by downregulation of mgmt in t98g glioblastoma cells by the nf-kappab-dependent pathway. *Oncol. Rep.* **2012**, *27*, 2050–2056. [PubMed]
52. Yang, H.C.; Wang, J.Y.; Bu, X.Y.; Yang, B.; Wang, B.Q.; Hu, S.; Yan, Z.Y.; Gao, Y.S.; Han, S.Y.; Qu, M.Q. Resveratrol restores sensitivity of glioma cells to temozolamide through inhibiting the activation of wnt signaling pathway. *J. Cell. Physiol.* **2018**, *2018*. [CrossRef]
53. Koval, A.; Katanaev, V.L. Dramatic dysbalancing of the wnt pathway in breast cancers. *Sci. Rep.* **2018**, *8*, 7329. [CrossRef] [PubMed]
54. Zhu, Y.; He, W.; Gao, X.; Li, B.; Mei, C.; Xu, R.; Chen, H. Resveratrol overcomes gefitinib resistance by increasing the intracellular gefitinib concentration and triggering apoptosis, autophagy and senescence in pc9/g nsclc cells. *Sci. Rep* **2015**, *5*, 17730. [CrossRef] [PubMed]
55. Li, W.; Ma, X.; Li, N.; Liu, H.; Dong, Q.; Zhang, J.; Yang, C.; Liu, Y.; Liang, Q.; Zhang, S.; et al. Resveratrol inhibits hexokinases ii mediated glycolysis in non-small cell lung cancer via targeting akt signaling pathway. *Exp. Cell Res.* **2016**, *349*, 320–327. [CrossRef]
56. Wang, J.; Li, J.; Cao, N.; Li, Z.; Han, J.; Li, L. Resveratrol, an activator of sirt1, induces protective autophagy in non-small-cell lung cancer via inhibiting akt/mtor and activating p38-mapk. *OncoTargets Ther.* **2018**, *11*, 7777–7786. [CrossRef] [PubMed]
57. Ahmad, A.; Gadgeel, S.M. Lung cancer and personalized medicine: Novel therapies and clinical management. Preface. *Adv. Exp. Med. Biol.* **2016**, *890*, v–vi.
58. Ahmad, A. Epigenetics in personalized management of lung cancer. *Adv Exp Med Biol* **2016**, *890*, 111–122.
59. Fudhaili, A.; Yoon, N.A.; Kang, S.; Ryu, J.; Jeong, J.Y.; Lee, D.H.; Kang, S.S. Resveratrol epigenetically regulates the expression of zinc finger protein 36 in nonsmall cell lung cancer cell lines. *Oncol. Rep.* **2019**, *41*, 1377–1386.
60. Gupta, G.; Bebawy, M.; Pinto, T.J.A.; Chellappan, D.K.; Mishra, A.; Dua, K. Role of the tristetraprolin (zinc finger protein 36 homolog) gene in cancer. *Crit. Rev. Eukaryot. Gene. Expr.* **2018**, *28*, 217–221. [CrossRef]
61. Howitz, K.T.; Bitterman, K.J.; Cohen, H.Y.; Lamming, D.W.; Lavu, S.; Wood, J.G.; Zipkin, R.E.; Chung, P.; Kisielewski, A.; Zhang, L.L.; et al. Small molecule activators of sirtuins extend saccharomyces cerevisiae lifespan. *Nature* **2003**, *425*, 191–196. [CrossRef] [PubMed]
62. Venturelli, S.; Berger, A.; Bocker, A.; Busch, C.; Weiland, T.; Noor, S.; Leischner, C.; Schleicher, S.; Mayer, M.; Weiss, T.S.; et al. Resveratrol as a pan-hdac inhibitor alters the acetylation status of histone [corrected] proteins in human-derived hepatoblastoma cells. *PLoS ONE* **2013**, *8*, e73097.
63. Dutra, L.A.; Heidenreich, D.; Silva, G.; Man Chin, C.; Knapp, S.; Santos, J.L.D. Dietary compound resveratrol is a pan-bet bromodomain inhibitor. *Nutrients* **2017**, *9*, 1172. [CrossRef] [PubMed]
64. Sahni, J.M.; Keri, R.A. Targeting bromodomain and extraterminal proteins in breast cancer. *Pharmacol. Res.* **2018**, *129*, 156–176. [CrossRef] [PubMed]
65. Garmpis, N.; Damaskos, C.; Garmpi, A.; Kalampokas, E.; Kalampokas, T.; Spartalis, E.; Daskalopoulou, A.; Valsami, S.; Kontos, M.; Nonni, A.; et al. Histone deacetylases as new therapeutic targets in triple-negative breast cancer: Progress and promises. *Cancer Genom. Proteom.* **2017**, *14*, 299–313.
66. Damaskos, C.; Garmpis, N.; Valsami, S.; Kontos, M.; Spartalis, E.; Kalampokas, T.; Kalampokas, E.; Athanasiou, A.; Moris, D.; Daskalopoulou, A.; et al. Histone deacetylase inhibitors: An attractive therapeutic strategy against breast cancer. *Anticancer Res.* **2017**, *37*, 35–46. [CrossRef]
67. Zucchetti, B.; Shimada, A.K.; Katz, A.; Curigliano, G. The role of histone deacetylase inhibitors in metastatic breast cancer. *The Breast* **2018**, *43*, 130–134. [CrossRef] [PubMed]
68. Guo, P.; Chen, W.; Li, H.; Li, M.; Li, L. The histone acetylation modifications of breast cancer and their therapeutic implications. *Pathol. Oncol. Res.* **2018**, *24*, 807–813. [CrossRef]
69. Lee, H.; Zhang, P.; Herrmann, A.; Yang, C.; Xin, H.; Wang, Z.; Hoon, D.S.; Forman, S.J.; Jove, R.; Riggs, A.D.; et al. Acetylated stat3 is crucial for methylation of tumor-suppressor gene promoters and inhibition by resveratrol results in demethylation. *Proc. Natl. Acad. Sci. USA* **2012**, *109*, 7765–7769. [CrossRef]
70. Lapidus, R.G.; Nass, S.J.; Butash, K.A.; Parl, F.F.; Weitzman, S.A.; Graff, J.G.; Herman, J.G.; Davidson, N.E. Mapping of er gene cpg island methylation-specific polymerase chain reaction. *Cancer Res.* **1998**, *58*, 2515–2519.

71. Saenglee, S.; Jogloy, S.; Patanothai, A.; Leid, M.; Senawong, T. Cytotoxic effects of peanut phenolics possessing histone deacetylase inhibitory activity in breast and cervical cancer cell lines. *Pharmacol. Rep.* **2016**, *68*, 1102–1110. [PubMed]
72. Parashar, G.; Capalash, N. Promoter methylation-independent reactivation of pax1 by curcumin and resveratrol is mediated by uhrf1. *Clin. Exp. Med.* **2016**, *16*, 471–478. [CrossRef] [PubMed]
73. Beyer, S.; Zhu, J.; Mayr, D.; Kuhn, C.; Schulze, S.; Hofmann, S.; Dannecker, C.; Jeschke, U.; Kost, B.P. Histone h3 acetyl k9 and histone h3 tri methyl k4 as prognostic markers for patients with cervical cancer. *Int. J. Mol. Sci.* **2017**, *18*, 477. [CrossRef] [PubMed]
74. Plewka, D.; Plewka, A.; Miskiewicz, A.; Morek, M.; Bogunia, E. Nuclear factor-kappa b as potential therapeutic target in human colon cancer. *J. Cancer Res. Ther.* **2018**, *14*, 516–520. [CrossRef]
75. Pu, J.; Bai, D.; Yang, X.; Lu, X.; Xu, L.; Lu, J. Adrenaline promotes cell proliferation and increases chemoresistance in colon cancer ht29 cells through induction of mir-155. *Biochem. Biophys. Res. Commun.* **2012**, *428*, 210–215. [CrossRef] [PubMed]
76. Jung, Y.J.; Lee, J.E.; Lee, A.S.; Kang, K.P.; Lee, S.; Park, S.K.; Lee, S.Y.; Han, M.K.; Kim, D.H.; Kim, W. Sirt1 overexpression decreases cisplatin-induced acetylation of nf-kappab p65 subunit and cytotoxicity in renal proximal tubule cells. *Biochem. Biophys. Res. Commun.* **2012**, *419*, 206–210. [CrossRef] [PubMed]
77. Buhrmann, C.; Shayan, P.; Popper, B.; Goel, A.; Shakibaei, M. Sirt1 is required for resveratrol-mediated chemopreventive effects in colorectal cancer cells. *Nutrients* **2016**, *8*, 145. [CrossRef]
78. Yaseen, A.; Chen, S.; Hock, S.; Rosato, R.; Dent, P.; Dai, Y.; Grant, S. Resveratrol sensitizes acute myelogenous leukemia cells to histone deacetylase inhibitors through reactive oxygen species-mediated activation of the extrinsic apoptotic pathway. *Mol. Pharmacol.* **2012**, *82*, 1030–1041. [CrossRef]
79. Frazzi, R.; Valli, R.; Tamagnini, I.; Casali, B.; Latruffe, N.; Merli, F. Resveratrol-mediated apoptosis of hodgkin lymphoma cells involves sirt1 inhibition and foxo3a hyperacetylation. *Int. J. Cancer* **2013**, *132*, 1013–1021. [CrossRef]
80. Kikuchi, H.; Mimuro, H.; Kuribayashi, F. Resveratrol strongly enhances the retinoic acid-induced superoxide generating activity via up-regulation of gp91-phox gene expression in u937 cells. *Biochem. Biophys. Res. Commun.* **2018**, *495*, 1195–1200. [CrossRef]
81. Kai, L.; Samuel, S.K.; Levenson, A.S. Resveratrol enhances p53 acetylation and apoptosis in prostate cancer by inhibiting mta1/nurd complex. *Int. J. Cancer* **2010**, *126*, 1538–1548. [CrossRef] [PubMed]
82. Xue, Y.; Wong, J.; Moreno, G.T.; Young, M.K.; Cote, J.; Wang, W. Nurd, a novel complex with both atp-dependent chromatin-remodeling and histone deacetylase activities. *Mol. Cell* **1998**, *2*, 851–861. [CrossRef]
83. Li, K.; Dias, S.J.; Rimando, A.M.; Dhar, S.; Mizuno, C.S.; Penman, A.D.; Lewin, J.R.; Levenson, A.S. Pterostilbene acts through metastasis-associated protein 1 to inhibit tumor growth, progression and metastasis in prostate cancer. *PLoS ONE* **2013**, *8*, e57542. [CrossRef] [PubMed]
84. Dhar, S.; Kumar, A.; Li, K.; Tzivion, G.; Levenson, A.S. Resveratrol regulates pten/akt pathway through inhibition of mta1/hdac unit of the nurd complex in prostate cancer. *Biochim. Biophys. Acta* **2015**, *1853*, 265–275. [CrossRef] [PubMed]
85. Harada, N.; Atarashi, K.; Murata, Y.; Yamaji, R.; Nakano, Y.; Inui, H. Inhibitory mechanisms of the transcriptional activity of androgen receptor by resveratrol: Implication of DNA binding and acetylation of the receptor. *J. Steroid Biochem. Mol. Biol.* **2011**, *123*, 65–70. [CrossRef]
86. Chao, S.C.; Chen, Y.J.; Huang, K.H.; Kuo, K.L.; Yang, T.H.; Huang, K.Y.; Wang, C.C.; Tang, C.H.; Yang, R.S.; Liu, S.H. Induction of sirtuin-1 signaling by resveratrol induces human chondrosarcoma cell apoptosis and exhibits antitumor activity. *Sci. Rep.* **2017**, *7*, 3180. [CrossRef]
87. Zadi Heydarabad, M.; Nikasa, M.; Vatanmakanian, M.; Azimi, A.; Farshdousti Hagh, M. Regulatory effect of resveratrol and prednisolone on mdr1 gene expression in acute lymphoblastic leukemia cell line (ccrf-cem): An epigenetic perspective. *J. Cell Biochem.* **2018**, *119*, 4890–4896. [CrossRef]

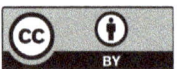

© 2019 by the authors. Licensee MDPI, Basel, Switzerland. This article is an open access article distributed under the terms and conditions of the Creative Commons Attribution (CC BY) license (http://creativecommons.org/licenses/by/4.0/).

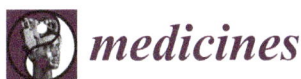

Review

The Multitarget Activity of Natural Extracts on Cancer: Synergy and Xenohormesis

María Herranz-López, María Losada-Echeberría and Enrique Barrajón-Catalán *

Instituto de Biología Molecular y Celular (IBMC) and Instituto de Investigación, Desarrollo e Innovación en Biotecnología Sanitaria de Elche (IDiBE), Universitas Miguel Hernández 03202 Elche, Spain; mherranz@umh.es (M.H.-L.); mlosada@umh.es (M.L.-E.)
* Correspondence: e.barrajon@umh.es; Tel.: +34-965-222-586

Received: 30 November 2018; Accepted: 24 December 2018; Published: 28 December 2018

Abstract: It is estimated that over 60% of the approved drugs and new drug developments for cancer and infectious diseases are from natural origin. The use of natural compounds as a potential source of antitumor agents has been deeply studied in many cancer models, both in vitro and in vivo. Most of the Western medicine studies are based on the use of highly selective pure compounds with strong specificity for their targets such as colchicine or taxol. Nevertheless, approximately 60% of fairly specific drugs in their initial research fail because of toxicity or ineffectiveness in late-stage preclinical studies. Moreover, cancer is a multifaceted disease that in most cases deserves a polypharmacological therapeutic approach. Complex plant-derived mixtures such as natural extracts are difficult to characterize and hardly exhibit high pharmacological potency. However, in some cases, these may provide an advantage due to their multitargeted mode of action and potential synergistic behavior. The polypharmacology approach appears to be a plausible explanation for the multigargeted mechanism of complex natural extracts on different proteins within the same signalling pathway and in several biochemical pathways at once. This review focuses on the different aspects of natural extracts in the context of anticancer activity drug development, with special attention to synergy studies and xenohormesis.

Keywords: cancer; natural compound; synergy; xenohormesis; polypharmacology

1. Introduction

Cancer is not a single disease, but a complex clinical situation in which multiple molecular pathways and cellular processes are compromised. Each cancer type has its own molecular fingerprint and, at least one of the cancer hallmarks described in [1], is altered. However, in spite of this heterogeneous situation, all cancers have a common behavior based on uncontrolled proliferation and invasion. This invasive phenotype is the real clinical problem and, in most cases, still remains unresolved, causing morbidity and mortality.

Anticancer research and drug discovery are continuously increasing the therapeutic arsenal, and relevant advances have been made towards individualized treatments [2–5]. New antibody-based drugs, called biological treatments [6,7], have improved treatments and prognosis in some cancer types such as breast, lung, liver cancers and lymphoma. New specific inhibitor families have also been developed, especially against proliferation related kinases. These drugs are called "inibs" [8,9]. In this sense, there is a tendency to look for highly specific drugs within the low micromolar range to solve very specific, almost individual cases. In vitro and in silico approaches have propelled the development of these specific drugs, and our bibliography is full of these examples [10–13]. These specific drugs follow the classic pharmacological dogma "one drug-one target", but in spite of their undeniable value, they lack some relevant aspects that will be discussed in the following sections.

On the contrary, the molecular promiscuity of some molecules, especially those from natural origin [14,15], allow them to exert a potential multitarget mechanism of action. These compounds are able to interact with different targets, modifying different pathways or different steps of the same signaling cascade. In addition, promiscuity is not always due to a single compound but a mixture of compounds, as occurs in some complex natural extracts. In these cases, each compound is able to interact with one or multiple targets, increasing the pharmacological promiscuity of the whole drug. In addition, natural extracts or their main components can be combined with conventional chemotherapy, reducing the development of resistance to antitumor drugs and toxic effects [16].

This review will be focused on discussing the advantages and drawbacks of the use of natural extracts when compared with classical individual targeting strategy. Xenohormesis, multitargeting, synergy and drug resistance will be the main points that will be addressed.

2. Natural Compounds, Hormesis and Xenohormesis

Chemistry and analytical advances have allowed the synthesis and characterization of millions of new molecules for drug discovery. In some cases, synthesis was structurally guided using in silico or structural approaches, in others, combinatorial libraries were built based on a molecular scaffold or leads. This approach has allowed the development of new drugs not only for cancer treatment but also for other diseases. However, all these drugs have been human-designed and lack natural origin. On the contrary, natural extracts and their compounds have been selected for by millions of years of evolution as complex sources of medicinal agents. This is the basis of xenohormesis hypothesis [17,18]. They present very diverse chemical structures, from the simplest phenolic acids in plants to the most complex marine compounds [19–21]. Glycosylation, methylation and other esterifications and the presence of other moieties, increase the number and diversity of natural compounds. This constitutes a countless and invaluable source of new drugs. From a biomedical point of view, hormesis is an adaptive response in which the exposure to a low dose of an environmental factor or chemical compound, that is harmful at high concentrations, has a beneficial and/or adaptive effect on a cell or organism. Sometimes this response is mediated by some compounds that, when incorporated in the heterotroph diet, induce biological responses leading to pharmacological effects. This final effect is called xenohormesis, as the final benefit is obtained by the heterotroph organism, not for the plant that originally adapted to the stressful condition [17,18]. Xenohormesis is a way of cross-species interaction and communication.

Although hormesis is an essential concept in evolution, xenohormesis has also allowed the expansion and fixation of evolutionary advances in non-autotrophs organisms. Nowadays, xenohormesis gives us a chance to obtain benefits from natural compounds and obtain new drugs selected by nature all through the evolution process. These compounds can be used directly for anticancer drug discovery, and also as new leads in novel developments using the classical structurally guided or in silico approaches. This is one of the main advantages of natural extracts and their compounds. They can be used as any other drugs, but with the benefit of being selected by natural evolution.

3. Combined Therapies, Multitargeting and Synergy

Based on the classic pharmacological dogma "one drug-one target", monotherapy has been the traditional approach, not only to treat diseases, but also to find new active drugs against a chosen target. However, presently there is evidence pointing out that combined therapies are much more efficient than single-drug-based treatments. In this sense, combinational therapy is extended to treat not only cancer but also other diseases, such as AIDS, bacterial infections, hypertension, metabolic or rheumatic disorders [22].

Combined drug therapy design is a hard and challenging task. Individual and combined actions must be characterized and it sometimes requires new preclinical and clinical trials. In addition, these multiple comparisons are sometimes difficult to incorporate into those studies.

Combined therapies are normally based on co-administration of two or more drugs. These combined drugs can be based on the combination of pure compounds, or can be achieved by using drugs based on mixtures of natural extracts.

Combined therapies are based on targeting different molecular signatures of the disease. On the one hand, multitargeting makes drug screening more complicated as complex assays must be developed to test all possibilities. On the other hand, multitargeting creates the opportunity to obtain synergic interactions between the combined therapy elements and drug resistance development, as detailed in further sections. There is a plethora of combined chemotherapy treatments covering most of the different cancer phenotypes. In fact, most of the recommended treatment regimens include two or more drugs, but as mentioned above, combined therapy use is not exclusive to cancer treatments, it is also extended to other disciplines such as antimicrobial and antihypertensive diseases.

Synergy is therefore the most relevant characteristic of combined therapies, including natural extracts. The first impetus for synergy research came from pharmaceutical legislation which demands the verification that every compound of a combined pharmaceutical preparation contributes to the claimed complete efficacy [22]. In terms of pharmacology, synergy is the ability of some mixtures to be more potent than the sum of their individual components. This definition is exportable to other disciplines and is based on the complementary as well as additive mechanism of action. Accordingly, synergy is not an absolute factor and the pharmacological interaction between the components of a mixture can be more or less synergic. This aspect is the main difference between additive and synergic behavior and is sometimes forgotten by researchers and clinicians.

Another aspect to be analyzed is that a single mixture is able to perform in a different way depending on the proportion of its components. According to this, different proportions of the same compounds could provide different results in terms of synergy, not only in an absolute way, but also in terms of being more or less synergic [23]. In this sense, an ideal proportion which provides the highest synergy results is always mathematically possible.

There are several ways to develop synergy studies, but in all cases, a previous and detailed design is required to obtain conclusive results. Most synergy studies fail because of a deficient design, both in qualitative and quantitative ways. There are several exhaustive and relevant reviews on synergy [22,24–26], so this review will not go deeper into how to study it. However, some aspects about study design deserve a comment:

- Drug selection: The right selection of the drugs for synergy studies is the first step to succeed. There are multiple available drugs for a single disease, but not all are suitable for a synergy study. Drugs must be selected considering different molecular targets. If not, antagonism or other undesired pharmacological interactions can be obtained. These different molecular targets can be located in different molecules, in distinguished epitopes of the same molecule or even in molecules of different pathways.
- Synergy study method: As mentioned above, there are several methods to study synergy between drugs. Quantitative methods such as Combination Index (CI) [27] or Fractional Inhibitory Concentration Index (FICI) [14] calculation are preferred as they obtain better conclusions.
- Biological assay: According to the selected method for synergy studies, a robust and reliable biological assay must be selected that allows testing a high number of samples with a large variability in composition. Survival or viability tests are diverse and allow high throughput screening approaches [28]. They are commonly used for anticancer compound research, but also for most of the other areas of drug discovery in which synergy is topical, such as antimicrobial drug discovery.
- Sample testing: Once the test is selected, an adequate design of the plates is also crucial. Checkboard plate design is probably the best approach for pairwise combinations using multi-wells plates. This strategy can be used not only for pairwise combinations but also for 3-drug combinations as shown in Figure 1.

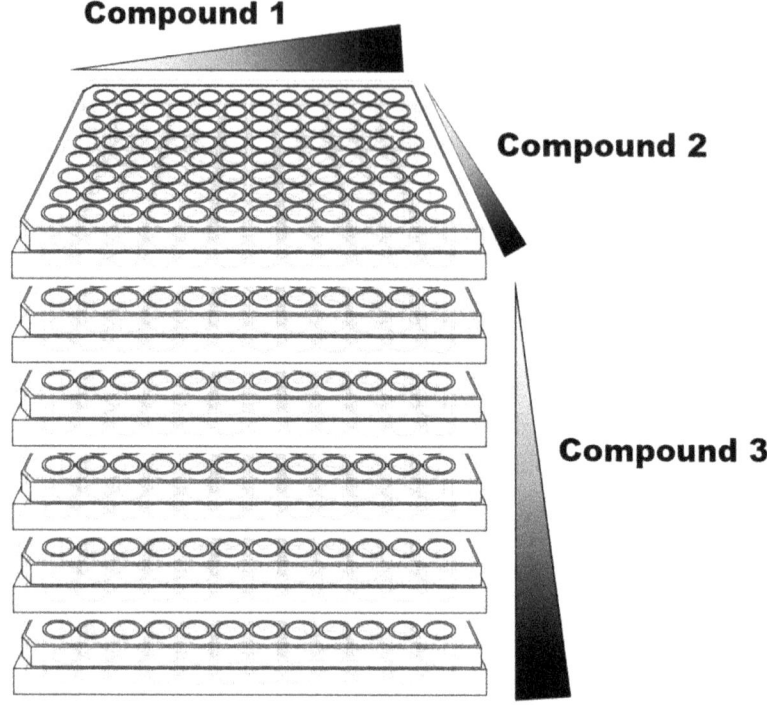

Figure 1. Checkboard plate design can be used not only for single plate experiments but also for more complex studies using three different compounds. In these cases, the concentration of each compound increases in one of the three dimensions (x, y and z axis) as indicated in the figure.

Following these recommendations, the final results will not only be scientifically relevant, but also comparable to other single drug or combined therapies. This will allow researchers and clinicians to obtain better conclusions and contribute to the development of new therapeutic approaches.

4. Examples of Synergy Studies

References to synergic interactions between drugs in cancer research are abundant in the bibliography. However, focusing on natural extract synergy studies, three main groups of examples can be classified. The first group includes studies covering complex extracts whose components present synergistic interactions among them. The second group includes examples of synergy between different extracts and natural compounds of different origin. Finally, the third group comprises examples of anticancer approved drugs combined with natural compounds or extracts. Some of the most relevant examples of each category are listed below and shown in Table 1.

Table 1. Examples of synergic interactions among compounds or compounds and approved drugs in cancer research. Main examples included in this manuscript are shown in this table, organized in rows. First and second columns indicate the name of the components among which synergy is obtained. Third and fourth and fifth columns show the cellular models in which synergy studies were performed (including their origin), the main effect and the bibliographic reference.

Extract/Compound	Synergy	Experimental Model (Cell Line)	Effect	References
Pomegranate extract	Among their compounds	Oral cancer (KB, CAL27), colon cancer (HT-29, HCT116, SW480, SW620) and prostate cancer (RWPE-1, 22Rv1)	Antiproliferative, apoptotic and antioxidant	[29]
Pomegranate extract	Among their compounds	Prostate cancer (DU 145)	Antiproliferative, antimetastatic and phospholipase A2 (PLA2) inhibition	[30]
Grape extract	Among their compounds and with Ara-C and tazofurin	Leukemia (HL-60)	Antiproliferative and apoptotic	[31]
Grape extract	Among their compounds	Colon cancer (HCT116)	Antiproliferative and apoptotic	[32]
Rosemary extract	Among their compounds	Colon cancer (HT-29)	Antiproliferative	[33]
Ginger extract	Among their compounds	Prostate cancer (PC-3)	Antiproliferative	[34]
Graviola flavonoids	Among their compounds	Prostate cancer (PC-3)	Antiproliferative	[35]
Turmeric extract	With rosemary compounds	Breast cancer (MDA-MB-453, MDA-MB-468, and MCF7)	Antiproliferative, G1 cell cycle arrest	[36]
Tea extract	With capsicum compounds	Cervical cancer (HeLa) and breast cancer (4T1)	Antiproliferative	[37]
Tea extract	With soy compounds	Mice *in vivo* model	Metabolic effect	[38]
Tea extract	With soy compounds	Prostate cancer (LnCAP) xenotrasplants	Antiproliferative	[39]
Tea extract	With others tea extracts	Review	Antioxidant, antimicrobial and antitumoral	[40]
Resveratrol	With quercetin and ellagic acid	Leukemia (MOLT-4)	Antiproliferative, apoptosis and cel cycle arrest	[41,42]
Carothenoids	With other phytochemicals	Prostate cancer LNCaP, PC-3 and DU-145) and breast cancer (MCF-7)	Antiproliferative	[43]
Genistein	With cisplatin, 5-fluorouracil, arsenic trioxide, doxorubicin, gemcitabine camptothecine and hidroxi-camptothecine	Pancreatic cancer (BxPC-3 xenograft, COL-357 and L3.6pl) colon cancer (HT29), hepatic cancer (HepG2, Hep3B, SK-Hep-1, HEpG2 xenograft), cervical cancer (HeLa) ovarian cancer (OAW-42), bladder cancer (TCC-SUP) and lung cancer (ME-180pt, UMSCC-5)	Antiproliferative	[44]
Curcumin	With 5-fluorouracil, oxaliplatin, cisplatin, etoposide, camptothecine and doxorubicine	Colon cancer (HT-29), ovarian cancer (2008 and C13) and human and rat glioblastoma cell lines	Antiproliferative	[44]
(-)-epigallocatechin-3-gallate	With doxorubicin, gemcitabine and cisplatin	Carcinoma doxorubicin resistant (KB-A-1 xenograft), cholangiocarcinoma (Mz-ChA-1 cell line and xenograft) and ovarian cancer (SKOC3, CAOV3 and C200)	Antiproliferative	[44]
Quercetin	With doxorubicin, cisplatin, arsenic trioxide and temozolomide	Neuroblastoma and Edwing's sarcoma cell lines, laryngeal cancer (Hep2), leukemia (U937 and HL-60) and astrocytoma	Antiproliferative	[44]
Resveratrol	With Cisplatin and doxorubicin	Acute leukemia (ML-2/DX30, AML-2/DX100 and AML-2/DX300)	Antiproliferative	[44]

Pomegranate polyphenolic extracts have demonstrated numerous biological activities such as antioxidant, cardiovascular preventive and antitumoral activities [45–48]. These extracts are enriched in ellagitannins such as ellagic acid, punicalagin and punicalin. Synergy studies between pomegranate polyphenols have been performed in colon cancer cells [29], prostate [30] and other cellular models [49]. Grape fruit is also a well-known source of active compounds, including resveratrol as the most representative one. As with pomegranate, grape extracts present abundant biological activities [31,50]. In regards to cancer and synergy studies, grape polyphenols have shown synergy between them, especially on colon cancer cell models [32]. Rosemary terpenes have also shown antitumoral synergic activity on colon cancer cells [33]. Ginger compounds [34], graviola flavonoids and acetogenin's action on prostate cancer [35] are examples of synergic interactions between different compounds included those that are present in the same extract.

In addition to single complex natural extracts, some studies have tested the synergic interactions between different extracts and/or different natural compounds, even mixing a complex natural extract with an individual natural compound. On the one hand, turmeric extracts have showed synergic activity with rosemary extracts as well as their representative compounds, carnosic acid and curcumin [36]. Tea natural compounds, mainly catechins, synergistically interact with capsicum compounds [37], soy phytochemicals [38,39] and between different tea extracts [40]. On the other hand, individual compounds such as resveratrol, quercetin and ellagic acid also interact synergistically in human leukemia cells [41,42]. Carotenoids and other phytochemicals also presented similar behavior [43]. Finally, natural compounds and extracts synergistically interact with clinically used anticancer drugs as occurs between many polyphenols and anticancer drugs such as cisplatin, doxorubicin, 5-fluoracil and others as reviewed in Reference [44].

5. Drawbacks of Using Natural Compounds

Pure natural compounds have demonstrated the same validity as synthetic or semisynthetic drugs in drug discovery. They are single compounds with a well-known chemical structure. They can be obtained from natural resources, in most cases using synthetic or semisynthetic approaches [51,52]. However, natural extracts, regardless of vegetal, microorganism or animal origin, are usually complex mixtures. Two main consequences are derived from natural extract's complexity. First, these mixtures must be chemically characterized as much as possible. The improvement of analytical techniques such as liquid and gas chromatography coupled to mass detection, magnetic resonance and other approaches have permitted the characterization of very complex extracts [23,53–55]. The second consequence is that natural extract reproducibility is sometimes difficult due to the biological diversity of samples. This depends on origin, climate conditions, storage and extraction procedures. However, as occurred in other disciplines, this drawback can be avoided by controlling crop conditions, origin and extract production.

Natural compound bioavailability is also a drawback that deserves attention. Natural compounds have very different structures and, therefore, their bioavailability depend on the individual compound [56–58]. On the one hand, some natural compounds are quickly and fully absorbed, reaching the plasma in their native form so providing significant plasmatic concentrations. On the other hand, other natural compounds have scarce absorption, high metabolized rates and a fast excretion process. In all these cases, plasmatic concentration are low and biological activities are difficult to infer. Some strategies have been developed to improve natural compound bioavailability. Such as the use of different forms of encapsulation [59]; as nanoparticles [60,61], emulsion [62] or liposomes [63]. These approaches have been used especially to increase the solubility of highly hydrophobic compounds and extracts, and to improve the bioavailability of hydrophilic compounds with low stability or poor absorption [64,65]. However, in the end, natural compounds are not quite as different to other drugs that also present bioavailability limitations, and each case must be studied independently taking in account its solubility and the ADME processes.

Drug resistance is probably the most important problem of cancer treatments. There are many drug resistance mechanisms [66,67] and no drug is free to develop a resistant phenotype. Once again, natural compounds and extracts are not different to other drugs, and resistance phenomena may also take place. Combined therapies minimize the risk of drug resistance, as tumor cells that develops resistance against one of the drugs may be affected by other drugs or compounds present in the same mixture. In this sense, natural pure compounds perform as any other drug and can be used in combination to reduce resistance, but natural extracts are mixtures that may act as a combined therapy itself, contributing to a decrease in drug-resistant phenotypes.

6. Concluding Remarks

The current state of the art shows that combined therapies using natural extracts or combination of natural compounds and polypharmacology are quite promising. This is due to both the synergic interactions between their components and the reduction of drug resistant phenotype risk. Natural extracts are naturally occurring mixtures that have been selected by hormesis processes that can be beneficial to humans according to xenohormesis theory. They are indeed real combined therapies that, if well selected and characterized, can be used for new anticancer drugs development. In this sense, the design of high-quality synergy studies is crucial and a supplementary effort in this sense is worthy.

But not everything may be considered an advantage when using natural extracts, they share some drawbacks with conventional anticancer drugs. Poor bioavailability and drug resistance mechanisms are as common among natural extracts as with conventional drugs. However, the polypharmacological properties of natural extracts makes resistance more difficult and, as occurred with other conventional drugs, bioavailability problems can be addressed using different approaches such as encapsulation. The most important disadvantage of natural extracts is their complexity and reproducibility, but as mentioned above, technical advances and quality controls during processing can overcome this problem.

In conclusion, natural extracts are a promising source of new anticancer drugs, but also suppose a challenging issue. As in the past, natural extracts will continue to be used as sources to develop new anticancer agents. These compounds have been selected on an evolutionary basis that may suppose an advantage for their performance.

Nevertheless, the same criteria for safety, efficacy and quality that are required for their synthetic counterparts must be expected. Strong efforts must be applied in extract characterization and in synergy studies. Despite these challenges, natural extracts are an irreplaceable source of new anticancer compounds that undoubtedly will allow the development of new anticancer therapies in the future.

Funding: This research was funded by projects AGL2015-67995-C3-1-R, AGL2015-67995-C3-2-R and AGL2015-67995-C3-3-R from the Spanish Ministry of Economy and Competitiveness (MINECO); and PROMETEO/2012/007, PROMETEO/2016 ACIF/2010/162, ACIF/2015/158, ACIF/2016/230 and APOSTD/2017/023 grants from *Generalitat Valenciana*.

Acknowledgments: Authors want to thank their lab supervisor, Vicente Micol, for his invaluable support.

Conflicts of Interest: The authors declare no conflict of interest.

References

1. Hanahan, D.; Weinberg, R.A. Hallmarks of cancer: The next generation. *Cell* **2011**, *144*, 646–674. [CrossRef] [PubMed]
2. Diamandis, M.; White, N.M.A.; Yousef, G.M. Personalized medicine: Marking a new epoch in cancer patient management. *Mol. Cancer Res.* **2010**, *8*, 1175–1187. [CrossRef] [PubMed]
3. Jain, K.K. Personalized medicine. *Curr. Opin. Mol. Ther.* **2002**, *4*, 548–558. [PubMed]
4. Olopade, O.I.; Grushko, T.A.; Nanda, R.; Huo, D. Advances in breast cancer: Pathways to personalized medicine. *Clin. Cancer Res.* **2008**, *14*, 7988–7999. [CrossRef] [PubMed]
5. Wang, E.; Zaman, N.; McGee, S.; Milanese, J.S.; Masoudi-Nejad, A.; O'Connor-McCourt, M. Predictive genomics: A cancer hallmark network framework for predicting tumor clinical phenotypes using genome sequencing data. *Semin. Cancer Biol.* **2015**, *30*, 4–12. [CrossRef] [PubMed]
6. Scott, A.M.; Wolchok, J.D.; Old, L.J. Antibody therapy of cancer. *Nat. Rev. Cancer* **2012**, *12*, 278–287. [CrossRef] [PubMed]
7. Weiner, L.M.; Surana, R.; Wang, S. Monoclonal antibodies: Versatile platforms for cancer immunotherapy. *Nat. Rev. Immunol.* **2010**, *10*, 317–327. [CrossRef]
8. Lee, Y.T.; Tan, Y.J.; Oon, C.E. Molecular targeted therapy: Treating cancer with specificity. *Eur. J. Pharmacol.* **2018**, *834*, 188–196. [CrossRef]
9. Arora, A.; Scholar, E.M. Role of tyrosine kinase inhibitors in cancer therapy. *J. Pharmacol. Exp. Ther.* **2005**, *315*, 971–979. [CrossRef]
10. Edelman, L.B.; Eddy, J.A.; Price, N.D. In silico models of cancer. *Wiley Interdiscip. Rev. Syst. Biol. Med.* **2010**, *2*, 438–459. [CrossRef]

11. Ruiz-Torres, V.; Losada-Echeberría, M.; Herranz-López, M.; Barrajón-Catalán, E.; Galiano, V.; Micol, V.; Encinar, A.J. New Mammalian Target of Rapamycin (mTOR) Modulators Derived from Natural Product Databases and Marine Extracts by Using Molecular Docking Techniques. *Mar. Drugs* **2018**, *16*, 385. [CrossRef] [PubMed]
12. Bellamy, W.T. Prediction of Response to Drug Therapy of Cancer: A Review of In Vitro Assays. *Drugs* **1992**, *44*, 690–708. [CrossRef] [PubMed]
13. Nyga, A.; Cheema, U.; Loizidou, M. 3D tumour models: Novel in vitro approaches to cancer studies. *J. Cell Commun. Signal.* **2011**, *5*, 239–248. [CrossRef] [PubMed]
14. Barrajon-Catalan, E.; Herranz-Lopez, M.; Joven, J.; Segura-Carretero, A.; Alonso-Villaverde, C.; Menendez, J.A.; Micol, V. Molecular promiscuity of plant polyphenols in the management of age-related diseases: Far beyond their antioxidant properties. *Adv. Exp. Med. Biol.* **2014**, *824*, 141–159. [PubMed]
15. Joven, J.; Rull, A.; Rodriguez-Gallego, E.; Camps, J.; Riera-Borrull, M.; Hernández-Aguilera, A.; Martin-Paredero, V.; Segura-Carretero, A.; Micol, V.; Alonso-Villaverde, C.; et al. Multifunctional targets of dietary polyphenols in disease: A case for the chemokine network and energy metabolism. *Food Chem. Toxicol.* **2013**, *51*, 267–279. [CrossRef] [PubMed]
16. Rejhová, A.; Opattová, A.; Čumová, A.; Slíva, D.; Vodička, P. Natural compounds and combination therapy in colorectal cancer treatment. *Eur. J. Med. Chem.* **2018**, *144*, 582–594. [CrossRef] [PubMed]
17. Howitz, K.T.; Sinclair, D.A. Xenohormesis: Sensing the chemical cues of other species. *Cell* **2008**, *133*, 387–391. [CrossRef]
18. Menendez, J.A.; Joven, J.; Aragones, G.; Barrajon-Catalan, E.; Beltran-Debon, R.; Borras-Linares, I.; Camps, J.; Corominas-Faja, B.; Cufi, S.; Fernandez-Arroyo, S.; et al. Xenohormetic and anti-aging activity of secoiridoid polyphenols present in extra virgin olive oil: A new family of gerosuppressant agents. *Cell Cycle* **2013**, *12*, 555–578. [CrossRef]
19. Ruiz-Torres, V.; Encinar, J.; Herranz-López, M.; Pérez-Sánchez, A.; Galiano, V.; Barrajón-Catalán, E.; Micol, V. An Updated Review on Marine Anticancer Compounds: The Use of Virtual Screening for the Discovery of Small-Molecule Cancer Drugs. *Molecules* **2017**, *22*, 1037. [CrossRef]
20. Grochowski, D.M.; Skalicka-Wozniak, K.; Orhan, I.E.; Xiao, J.; Locatelli, M.; Piwowarski, J.P.; Granica, S.; Tomczyk, M. A comprehensive review of agrimoniin. *Ann. N. Y. Acad. Sci.* **2017**, *1401*, 166–180. [CrossRef]
21. Grochowski, D.M.; Locatelli, M.; Granica, S.; Cacciagrano, F.; Tomczyk, M. A Review on the Dietary Flavonoid Tiliroside. *Compr. Rev. Food Sci. Food Saf.* **2018**, *17*, 1395–1421. [CrossRef]
22. Wagner, H.; Ulrich-Merzenich, G. Synergy research: Approaching a new generation of phytopharmaceuticals. *Phytomedicine* **2009**, *16*, 97–110. [CrossRef] [PubMed]
23. Tomas-Menor, L.; Barrajon-Catalan, E.; Segura-Carretero, A.; Marti, N.; Saura, D.; Menendez, J.A.; Joven, J.; Micol, V. The promiscuous and synergic molecular interaction of polyphenols in bactericidal activity: An opportunity to improve the performance of antibiotics? *Phytother. Res.* **2015**, *29*, 466–473. [CrossRef] [PubMed]
24. Roell, K.R.; Reif, D.M.; Motsinger-Reif, A.A. An Introduction to Terminology and Methodology of Chemical Synergy-Perspectives from Across Disciplines. *Front. Pharmacol.* **2017**, *8*, 158. [CrossRef] [PubMed]
25. Chou, T.C. Drug combination studies and their synergy quantification using the chou-talalay method. *Cancer Res.* **2010**, *70*, 440–446. [CrossRef] [PubMed]
26. Greco, W.R.; Bravo, G.; Parsons, J.C. The search for synergy: A critical review from a response surface perspective. *Pharmacol. Rev.* **1995**, *47*, 331–385. [PubMed]
27. Chou, T.C. Theoretical basis, experimental design, and computerized simulation of synergism and antagonism in drug combination studies. *Pharmacol. Rev.* **2006**, *58*, 621–681. [CrossRef]
28. Stoddart, M.J. Cell viability assays: Introduction. *Methods Mol. Biol. (Clifton, N.J.)* **2011**, *740*, 1–6.
29. Seeram, N.P.; Adams, L.S.; Henning, S.M.; Niu, Y.; Zhang, Y.; Nair, M.G.; Heber, D. In vitro antiproliferative, apoptotic and antioxidant activities of punicalagin, ellagic acid and a total pomegranate tannin extract are enhanced in combination with other polyphenols as found in pomegranate juice. *J. Nutr. Biochem.* **2005**, *16*, 360–367. [CrossRef]
30. Lansky, E.P.; Jiang, W.; Mo, H.; Bravo, L.; Froom, P.; Yu, W.; Harris, N.M.; Neeman, I.; Campbell, M.J. Possible synergistic prostate cancer suppression by anatomically discrete pomegranate fractions. *Invest. New Drugs* **2005**, *23*, 11–20. [CrossRef]

31. Athar, M.; Back, J.H.; Tang, X.; Kim, K.H.; Kopelovich, L.; Bickers, D.R.; Kim, A.L. Resveratrol: A review of preclinical studies for human cancer prevention. *Toxicol. Appl. Pharmacol.* **2007**, *224*, 274–283. [CrossRef] [PubMed]
32. Radhakrishnan, S.; Reddivari, L.; Sclafani, R.; Das, U.N.; Vanamala, J. Resveratrol potentiates grape seed extract induced human colon cancer cell apoptosis. *Front. Biosci. Elite* **2011**, *3E*, 1509–1523. [CrossRef]
33. Pérez-Sánchez, A.; Barrajón-Catalán, E.; Ruiz-Torres, V.; Agulló-Chazarra, L.; Herranz-López, M.; Valdés, A.; Cifuentes, A.; Micol, V. Rosemary (Rosmarinus officinalis) extract causes ROS-induced necrotic cell death and inhibits tumor growth in vivo. *Sci. Rep.* **2018**. [CrossRef]
34. Brahmbhatt, M.; Gundala, S.R.; Asif, G.; Shamsi, S.A.; Aneja, R. Ginger phytochemicals exhibit synergy to inhibit prostate cancer cell proliferation. *Nutr. Cancer* **2013**, *65*, 263–272. [CrossRef] [PubMed]
35. Yang, C.; Gundala, S.R.; Mukkavilli, R.; Vangala, S.; Reid, M.D.; Aneja, R. Synergistic interactions among flavonoids and acetogenins in Graviola (Annona muricata) leaves confer protection against prostate cancer. *Carcinogenesis* **2015**, *36*, 656–665. [CrossRef] [PubMed]
36. Einbond, L.S.; Wu, H.A.; Kashiwazaki, R.; He, K.; Roller, M.; Su, T.; Wang, X.; Goldsberry, S. Carnosic acid inhibits the growth of ER-negative human breast cancer cells and synergizes with curcumin. *Fitoterapia* **2012**, *83*, 1160–1168. [CrossRef] [PubMed]
37. Morré, D.J.; Morré, D.M. Synergistic Capsicum-tea mixtures with anticancer activity. *J. Pharm. Pharmacol.* **2003**, *55*, 987–994. [CrossRef]
38. Zhou, J.R.; Li, L.; Pan, W. Dietary soy and tea combinations for prevention of breast and prostate cancers by targeting metabolic syndrome elements in mice. *Am. J. Clin. Nutr.* **2007**, *86*, 882S–888S. [CrossRef]
39. Zhou, J.R.; Yu, L.; Zhong, Y.; Blackburn, G.L. Soy phytochemicals and tea bioactive components synergistically inhibit androgen-sensitive human prostate tumors in mice. *J. Nutr.* **2003**, *133*, 516–521. [CrossRef]
40. Malongane, F.; McGaw, L.J.; Mudau, F.N. The synergistic potential of various teas, herbs and therapeutic drugs in health improvement: A review. *J. Sci. Food Agric.* **2017**, *97*, 4679–4689. [CrossRef]
41. Mertens-Talcott, S.U.; Percival, S.S. Ellagic acid and quercetin interact synergistically with resveratrol in the induction of apoptosis and cause transient cell cycle arrest in human leukemia cells. *Cancer Lett.* **2005**, *218*, 141–151. [CrossRef] [PubMed]
42. Mertens-Talcott, S.U.; Bomser, J.A.; Romero, C.; Talcott, S.T.; Percival, S.S. Ellagic acid potentiates the effect of quercetin on p21 waf1/cip1, p53, and MAP-kinases without affecting intracellular generation of reactive oxygen species in vitro. *J. Nutr.* **2005**, *135*, 609–614. [CrossRef] [PubMed]
43. Linnewiel-Hermoni, K.; Khanin, M.; Danilenko, M.; Zango, G.; Amosi, Y.; Levy, J.; Sharoni, Y. The anti-cancer effects of carotenoids and other phytonutrients resides in their combined activity. *Arch. Biochem. Biophys.* **2015**, *572*, 28–35. [CrossRef] [PubMed]
44. Lewandowska, U.; Gorlach, S.; Owczarek, K.; Hrabec, E.; Szewczyk, K. Synergistic interactions between anticancer chemotherapeutics and phenolic compounds and anticancer synergy between polyphenols. *Postepy Hig. Med. Dosw.* **2014**, *68*, 528–540. [CrossRef] [PubMed]
45. Basu, A.; Penugonda, K. Pomegranate juice: A heart-healthy fruit juice. *Nutr. Rev.* **2009**, *67*, 49–56. [CrossRef] [PubMed]
46. Bell, C.; Hawthorne, S. Ellagic acid, pomegranate and prostate cancer—A mini review. *J. Pharm. Pharmacol.* **2008**, *60*, 139–144. [CrossRef] [PubMed]
47. Landete, J.M. Ellagitannins, ellagic acid and their derived metabolites: A review about source, metabolism, functions and health. *Food Res. Int.* **2011**, *44*, 1150–1160. [CrossRef]
48. Larrosa, M.; García-Conesa, M.T.; Espín, J.C.; Tomás-Barberán, F.A. Ellagitannins, ellagic acid and vascular health. *Mol. Aspects Med.* **2010**, *31*, 513–539. [CrossRef]
49. Bishayee, A.; Bishayee, A. Pomegranate-derived constituents as inducers of cell death: Implications in cancer prevention and therapy. In *Natural Compounds as Inducers of Cell Death*; Springer: Dordrecht, The Netherlands, 2012; Volume 1, pp. 33–47.
50. Xia, E.Q.; Deng, G.F.; Guo, Y.J.; Li, H.B. Biological activities of polyphenols from grapes. *Int. J. Mol. Sci.* **2010**, *11*, 622–646. [CrossRef]
51. Herzon, S.B.; Vanderwal, C.D. Introduction: Natural Product Synthesis. *Chem. Rev.* **2017**, *117*, 11649–11650. [CrossRef]
52. Hale, K.J. (Ed.) *The Chemical Synthesis of Natural Products*; Willey: Hobolen, NJ, USA, 2000.

53. Barrajon-Catalan, E.; Fernandez-Arroyo, S.; Roldan, C.; Guillen, E.; Saura, D.; Segura-Carretero, A.; Micol, V. A systematic study of the polyphenolic composition of aqueous extracts deriving from several Cistus genus species: Evolutionary relationship. *Phytochem. Anal.* **2011**, *22*, 303–312. [CrossRef] [PubMed]
54. Borrás-Linares, I.; Herranz-López, M.; Barrajón-Catalán, E.; Arráez-Román, D.; González-Álvarez, I.; Bermejo, M.; Gutiérrez, A.F.; Micol, V.; Segura-Carretero, A. Permeability study of polyphenols derived from a phenolic-enriched hibiscus sabdariffa extract by UHPLC-ESI-UHR-Qq-TOF-MS. *Int. J. Mol. Sci.* **2015**, *16*, 18396–18411. [CrossRef] [PubMed]
55. Borrás-Linares, I.; Pérez-Sánchez, A.; Lozano-Sánchez, J.; Barrajón-Catalán, E.; Arráez-Román, D.; Cifuentes, A.; Micol, V.; Carretero, A.S. A bioguided identification of the active compounds that contribute to the antiproliferative/cytotoxic effects of rosemary extract on colon cancer cells. *Food Chem. Toxicol.* **2015**, *80*, 215–222. [CrossRef] [PubMed]
56. Olivares-Vicente, M.; Barrajón-Catalán, E.; Herranz-López, M.; Segura-Carretero, A.; Joven, J.; Encinar, J.A.; Micol, V. Plant-derived polyphenols in human health: Biological activity, metabolites and putative molecular targets. *Curr. Drug Metab.* **2018**, *19*, 351–369. [CrossRef] [PubMed]
57. D'Archivio, M.; Filesi, C.; Varì, R.; Scazzocchio, B.; Masella, R. Bioavailability of the polyphenols: Status and controversies. *Int. J. Mol. Sci.* **2010**, *11*, 1321–1342. [CrossRef] [PubMed]
58. Manach, C.; Scalbert, A.; Morand, C.; Rémésy, C.; Jiménez, L. Polyphenols: Food sources and bioavailability. *Am. J. Clin. Nutr.* **2004**, *79*, 727–747. [CrossRef] [PubMed]
59. Munin, A.; Edwards-Lévy, F. Encapsulation of natural polyphenolic compounds: A review. *Pharmaceutics* **2011**, *3*, 793–829. [CrossRef] [PubMed]
60. Khushnud, T.; Mousa, S.A. Potential role of naturally derived polyphenols and their nanotechnology delivery in cancer. *Mol. Biotechnol.* **2013**, *55*, 78–86. [CrossRef] [PubMed]
61. Liang, J.; Yan, H.; Puligundla, P.; Gao, X.; Zhou, Y.; Wan, X. Applications of chitosan nanoparticles to enhance absorption and bioavailability of tea polyphenols: A review. *Food Hydrocoll.* **2017**, *69*, 286–292. [CrossRef]
62. Lu, W.; Kelly, A.L.; Miao, S. Emulsion-based encapsulation and delivery systems for polyphenols. *Trends Food Sci. Technol.* **2016**, *47*, 1–9. [CrossRef]
63. Mignet, N.; Seguin, J.; Chabot, G.G. Bioavailability of polyphenol liposomes: A challenge ahead. *Pharmaceutics* **2013**, *5*, 457–471. [CrossRef] [PubMed]
64. Aditya, N.P.; Espinosa, Y.G.; Norton, I.T. Encapsulation systems for the delivery of hydrophilic nutraceuticals: Food application. *Biotechnol. Adv.* **2017**, *35*, 450–457. [CrossRef] [PubMed]
65. Barrajón-Catalán, E.; Funes, L.; Herranz-López, M.; González-Álvarez, I.; Bermejo, M.V.M. Differential absorption of curcuminoids between free and liposomed curcumin formulations. In *Curcumin: Clinical Uses, Health Effects and Potential Complications*; Martin, V., Ed.; Nova Publishers: Hauppauge, NY, USA, 2016; pp. 99–110.
66. Gottesman, M.M. Mechanisms of cancer drug resistance. *Annu. Rev. Med.* **2002**, *53*, 615–627. [CrossRef] [PubMed]
67. Mimeault, M.; Hauke, R.; Batra, S.K. Recent advances on the molecular mechanisms involved in the drug resistance of cancer cells and novel targeting therapies. *Clin. Pharmacol. Ther.* **2008**, *83*, 673–691. [CrossRef] [PubMed]

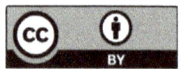

© 2018 by the authors. Licensee MDPI, Basel, Switzerland. This article is an open access article distributed under the terms and conditions of the Creative Commons Attribution (CC BY) license (http://creativecommons.org/licenses/by/4.0/).

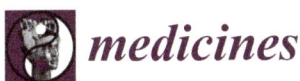

Review

Probiotics in the Treatment of Colorectal Cancer

Robert Hendler * and Yue Zhang

Department of Hematology and Oncology, Stony Brook University Hospital, Stony Brook,
New York, NY 11794, USA; yue.zhang@stonybrookmedicine.edu
* Correspondence: robert.hendler@stonybrookmedicine.edu; Tel.: +1-631-444-6000

Received: 20 August 2018; Accepted: 5 September 2018; Published: 7 September 2018

Abstract: The human microbiome plays many roles in inflammation, drug metabolism, and even the development of cancer that we are only beginning to understand. Colorectal cancer has been a focus for study in this field as its pathogenesis and its response to treatment have both been linked to the functioning of microbiota. This literature review evaluates the animal and human studies that have explored this relationship. By manipulating the microbiome with interventions such as probiotic administration, we may be able to reduce colorectal cancer risk and improve the safety and effectiveness of cancer therapy even though additional clinical research is still necessary.

Keywords: probiotics; synbiotics; microbiome; microbiota; colorectal cancer

1. Introduction

Globally, colorectal cancer is the third most commonly diagnosed type of cancer in men and the second most common in women [1]. In the United States, there are an estimated 135,430 new cases of colorectal cancer annually with an estimated 50,260 deaths due to the disease each year [2]. Colorectal cancer mortality has been improving over time in the United States by about 2.5% to 3% per year since 1990 [3] and while survival rates remain poor in advanced disease, early-stage colon cancer, this can potentially be cured with an estimated 74% five-year survival rate for patients with stage I disease [4]. As survival improves, it becomes more and more important to mitigate the adverse effects of colon cancer treatment. Surgery, chemotherapy, immune therapy, and radiation therapy all carry the possibility of significant treatment-related morbidity and mortality. In particular, adverse events affecting the gastrointestinal tract—such as nausea, diarrhea, colitis, and gastrointestinal bleeding—can diminish a patient's quality of life, preclude additional treatment, and sometimes even become life-threatening.

One promising avenue of study in the prevention and treatment of colorectal cancer is with the human microbiota. This refers to the 10 to 100 trillion symbiotic microbial cells harbored by each individual largely located in the gut where they are involved with metabolizing food remnants, intestinal and digestive secretions, and exfoliated colonocytes. The human microbiome, in turn, refers to the genes contained by these cells [5]. The microbiota serves a myriad of roles in the body with both positive and negative effects on human health and several large ongoing projects exist to explore this complex interplay [6,7]. Complicating this research is the fact that the microbiome is extremely diverse between individuals. The entire human genome consists of approximately 22,000 genes. This is compared to the human gut microbiome, which contains 3.3 million non-redundant genes that vary between individuals [5].

In the context of this diversity, there is debate over what makes up a "healthy" human microbiome. When the total DNA content of microbes inhabiting humans is analyzed, only one third of their constituent genes are found in a majority of healthy individuals [8]. Early research into the human microbiome had focused on identifying a core set of microbial taxa that were universally present in healthy people who lacked overt disease phenotypes on the assumption that certain specific microbes were essential to health. However, this proved to be an oversimplification as the variety of microbial species between individuals meant that characterizing an ideal set of specific microbes was not practical. An alternative hypothesis is that a healthy microbiome represents a "functional core"—a set of metabolic and other molecular functions performed by the microbiome that are not necessarily performed by the same organism in every individual.

As research into the microbiome progresses, we find that it affects health in ways we wouldn't expect. For instance, disruptions in the relative proportions of gut microbial populations may affect weight gain and insulin resistance contributing to type II diabetes mellitus [9]. These discoveries extend to the complex relationship between gut microflora, cancer development, and the effectiveness of cancer treatments. The composition of the microbiome has been correlated with colon cancer development in mouse [10,11] and human studies [12]. There is evidence that the effectiveness of various chemotherapy [13–15] and immune therapy [16,17] regimens depend on the composition of the microbiome.

Manipulating the microbiome using probiotics to improve the safety and GI side effect profile of cancer treatment has also been explored with a few studies evaluating the possible clinical benefit of probiotics with surgery [18], radiation therapy [19], and chemotherapy [20]. Probiotics are attractive as a potential complement to treatment because they are inexpensive and associated with few, if any, major adverse effects. Available evidence also suggests that probiotics may have a significant clinical impact. For instance, in one study of 168 patients evaluated after colorectal surgery for cancer, those receiving probiotics had a significantly decreased rate of all postoperative major complications when compared to the placebo arm (28.6% vs. 48.8%, $p = 0.010$) [21]. However, prospective studies evaluating the clinical effect of probiotics in cancer patients are currently few in number and more evidence is needed to determine the situations in which probiotics are beneficial.

In addition, the composition of the gut microbiome is heavily dependent on diet. In one mouse study, switching from a low-fat, plant polysaccharide-rich diet to a high-fat, high-sugar "Western" diet had major effects on the microbiome within one day with measurable changes in microbiome metabolic pathways and gene expression [22]. Of particular interest are prebiotics, which are non-digestible food ingredients that benefit the host by stimulating the growth or activity of commensal bacteria in the gut [23]. These have been shown to significantly change the microbiome composition. Administration of fructo-oligosaccharides, for instance, significantly increases the number of bifidobacteria found on fecal analysis and it decreases the amount of *Bacteroides*, *Fusobacteria*, and *Clostridium* [24]. Furthermore, prebiotics such as long and short chain oligosaccharides undergo fermentation in the colon by anaerobic bacteria, which metabolize them to short chain fatty acids (SCFAs) such as acetate, propionate, and butyrate. An increased concentration of SCFAs in the colon seems to have several beneficial effects including improved barrier function, increased intestinal mucus synthesis, stimulation of immunosuppressive cytokines such as interleukin 10 (IL-10), and reduced levels of pro-inflammatory mediators. Furthermore, increased SCFAs seem to result in the preferential growth of protective bacteria over pathogenic strains [25]. Synbiotics—combinations of pre-biotics and probiotics—have been shown to have similar beneficial regulatory effects.

2. Correlation between the Microbiome and Overall Gastrointestinal Health

We know from a number of studies that the microbiome plays an integral role in gastrointestinal health and function and that manipulation of the microbiome—using probiotics, for instance—can have beneficial effects (Figure 1). Commensal microorganisms exhibit mechanisms that appear to decrease inflammation. They combat pathogenic bacteria by producing bactericidal substances and competing with pathogens and toxins for adherence to the intestinal epithelium. Many regulate immune responses by enhancing innate immunity and modulating signaling pathways and others regulate intestinal epithelial homeostasis by promoting intestinal epithelial cell survival, enhancing barrier function, and stimulating cell protective responses [26]. Clinically, there have been a number of studies and meta-analyses showing a benefit of probiotics in a range of gastrointestinal diseases including pouchitis [27], infectious diarrhea [28,29], and chronic constipation [30]. Most of these studies have been small with methodological limitations. Due to differences in study composition, probiotic doses, and biological activity between various commercial probiotic preparations, results from any given study cannot be applied universally to all probiotic substances. Currently, no probiotic strategy represents standard of care or primary treatment for these GI issues. Nevertheless, given their potential benefit and anti-inflammatory properties, it stands to reason that probiotics may also have a beneficial effect in the prevention and treatment of cancer particularly with regard to preventing or alleviating the adverse effects of traditional cancer therapies.

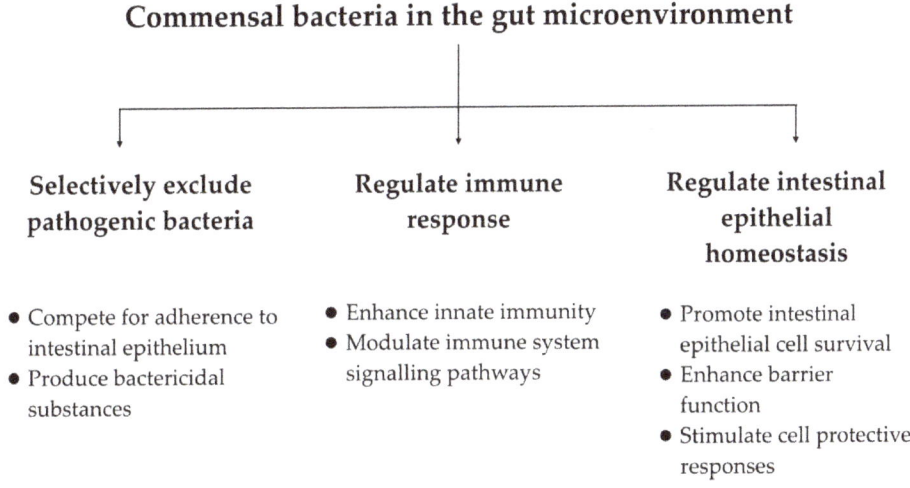

Figure 1. Proposed functions of gut commensal bacteria that may be beneficial in the prevention and treatment of colorectal cancer.

3. Correlation between the Microbiome and the Development of Colorectal Cancer

Recent research has shown that the composition of the microbiome in patients who have developed colorectal cancer is significantly different from the microbiome of patients who have not. A Japanese study that analyzed the micro-genome using terminal restriction fragment length polymorphism and next-generation sequencing analyses noted that several bacterial genera (*Actinomyces*, *Atopobium*, *Fusobacterium*, and *Haemophilus*) as well as several individual species (including *Bacteroides fragilis* and *Streptococcus gordonii*) were significantly associated with patients with known colorectal carcinoma but not in control patients without the disease [31]. Another study noted that microbiota close to the tumor tissue did not differ significantly when compared to the microbiota close to the normal mucosa in the same individual, which suggests that the microbiome does not change secondary to neoplasia but instead that colorectal cancer-distinctive microbiota may be present in the early stages of carcinogenesis [32]. We also know that dysbiosis—an imbalance or maladaptation of the microbiota—affects certain pathways that theoretically can lead to tumorigenesis [12] (Figure 2). Dysbiosis in the GI tract can lead to disruption of homeostasis of the immune system and mucosal barrier with subsequent inflammation resulting in increased mucosal barrier permeability and a continuous state of inflammation. This, in turn, can activate cytokines and growth factors such as tumor growth factor beta (TNF-β), tumor necrosis factor (TNF), IL-6, and vascular endothelial growth factor (VEGF), which can potentially lead to the growth and survival of dysplastic cells [33]. Dysbiosis with bacterial biofilm formation can also lead to increased bile acid metabolism, cell proliferation via Toll-like receptors, and other mechanisms that may, in turn, contribute to malignant transformation [34].

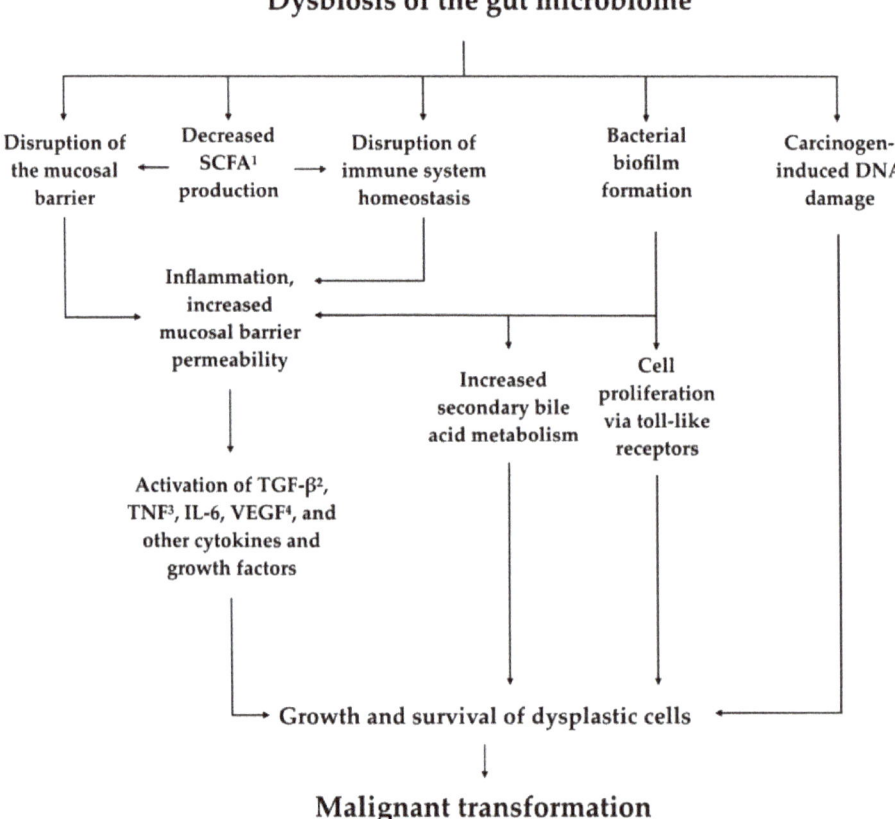

Figure 2. Overview of proposed mechanisms linking dysbiosis of the gut microbiome to tumorigenesis. [1] Short chain fatty acids. [2] Tumor growth factor beta. [3] Tumor necrosis factor. [4] Vascular endothelial growth factor.

Research into two types of bacteria called *Bacteroides fragilis* and *Fusobacterium nucleatum* provides models for how specific changes in the microbiome can contribute to tumorigenesis. A 2009 study examined enterotoxigenic *B. fragilis* (ETBF) and a cause of acute inflammatory diarrheal disease that also asymptomatically colonizes 20% to 35% of adults [35]. Both EBTF and nontoxigenic *B. fragilis* chronically colonized multiple intestinal neoplasia (Min) mice in the study, but only EBTF was shown to cause colitis and a strong induction of colonic tumors. It was found that ETBF activates the signal transducer and activates transcription-3 (Stat3) in the colon, which leads to colitis characterized by a T helper type 17 (T_H17) immune response. Antibody blockade of IL-17 and receptor of IL-23—key cytokines in the T_H17 response—was shown to inhibit the ETBF-induced colitis, subsequent colonic hyperplasia, and tumor formation.

Fusobacterium, particularly *F. nucleatum*, was shown to be over-represented in the genetic analysis of colorectal cancer tissue in two separate 2012 studies [36,37]. Prior to that, the species was linked to periodontitis and appendicitis but not to cancer. It was known that *F. nucleatum* could elicit a pro-inflammatory response, but it was initially unclear whether the bacteria contributed to tumorigenesis or if it was simply an opportunistic infection at the immunocompromised tumor site. Later on, mouse studies confirmed that *F. nucleatum* did, in fact, contribute to colorectal tumorigenesis and contribute to the stimulation of tumor cell growth by activating β-catenin signaling and inducing oncogenic gene expression by the FadA adhesion virulence factor [38].

Further studies on mouse models give us the strongest evidence that previously explored connections between dysbiosis and the development of malignancy are causative and not merely correlative. One study published in 2013 noted that tumor-bearing mice showed a different microbiome profile compared to non-tumor-bearing mice. When gut microbiota from tumor-bearing mice were introduced to and allowed to colonize germfree mice, the previously germfree mice were noted to have significantly increased tumorigenesis compared to mice that were colonized with microbiota from tumor-free mice. Furthermore, manipulation of the gut microbiome with antibiotics in these higher-risk mice resulted in a dramatic decrease in the number and size of tumors [11]. Another study in 2015 came to a similar conclusion by showing that isogenetic mice in a controlled environment exhibited different susceptibility to colorectal cancer depending on their distinct gut microflora profile [39].

4. Correlation between the Microbiome and Cancer Treatment Effectiveness

A major challenge in cancer therapy research is determining why certain patients will respond to a particular treatment while other patients with similar epidemiologic and clinical characteristics will not. A recent study has suggested that a patient's microbiome may play a much bigger role in response to systemic cancer therapy than previously realized. One recent *in vitro* study showed that exposing 5-FU-resistant colorectal cancer cells to *Lactobacillus plantarum* selectively inhibited characteristics of the cells including the expression of certain cancer-specific markers (CD44, 133, 166, and ALDH1). Treating the cells with combined *Lactobacillus plantarum* and 5-FU led to caspase-induced apoptosis and demonstrated further potential anticancer effects by inactivating the cells' Wnt/β-catenin signaling pathway [40]. In live subjects, mouse models have shown that disrupting the microbiota may decrease the effectiveness of systemic cancer therapies. One study evaluated mice that previously had received chronic treatment with antibiotics or were raised in a sterile environment. They were inoculated with subcutaneous tumors and given treatment with either an experimental immunotherapy (CpG-oligonucleotide) or platinum chemotherapy. Antibiotic-treated and germ-free mice had less cytokine production and very little tumor cell death after treatment with immunotherapy when compared to controls. When treated with platinum chemotherapy, the immune cells of antibiotic-treated and germ-free mice produced fewer of the enzymes necessary for generating reactive oxygen species [14]. A separate mouse study evaluated the relation between cyclophosphamide and microbiota. Cyclophosphamide was shown to induce certain Gram-positive bacteria to translocate from the small intestine to secondary lymphoid organs, which, in turn, stimulated a subset of helper and memory T-cells. Tumor-bearing mice that were antibiotic-treated or germ-free that did not have these specific bacteria showed reduced T-cell stimulation and a reduced tumor response after treatment with cyclophosphamide [41].

Other studies in mice have looked more specifically into how immunotherapy is affected by microbiota. The CTLA-4 blockade, for instance, appears to be dependent on T-cell responses specific for *Bacteroides thetaiotaomicron* or *Bacteroides fragilis*. In a 2015 study, it was found that tumors in antibiotic-treated or germ-free mice did not respond to treatment with a CTLA-4 blockade but that this lack of response could be overcome by gavage with *B. fragilis*. Interestingly, the CTLA-4 blockade was also found to be effective if *B. fragilis* polysaccharides were administered or if *B. fragilis*-specific T cells were transferred to the subject, which implies that the treatment's effectiveness was tied to the bacteria's stimulatory effect on the immune system and not to the continued presence of the bacteria itself. Furthermore, fecal microbial transplant from humans to mice showed that the treatment of melanoma patients with anti-CTLA-4 antibodies favored the outgrowth of *B. fragilis* with anticancer properties by affecting IL-12-dependent T-helper 1 (TH$_1$) immune responses to cancer [16]. A similar study done the same year compared melanoma growth in two groups of mice raised in two different facilities and known to harbor different populations of commensal bacteria. The groups showed differences in spontaneous antitumor immunity and tumor growth that disappeared after the mice from the two groups were housed together. Fecal transfer from mice in the population with less tumor growth to mice in the other population resulted in slower tumor growth as well as enhanced tumor infiltration with CD8 positive immune cells. Furthermore, anti-PD-L1 therapy was shown to be more effective in the lower-risk population of mice. Ribosomal RNA sequencing identified *Bifidobacterium* as being associated with antitumor effects. The researchers noted that oral administration of *Bifidobacterium* alone improved tumor control by the same amount as anti-PD-L1 therapy and that combining the two treatments "nearly abolished tumor outgrowth" in the mice [17].

While the results of these studies certainly cannot be directly applied to humans, they suggest that the effectiveness of many cancer therapies likely rely, at least in part, on the function of the microbiome. It is further speculated that this may mean the use of certain antibiotics may dampen the effect of certain anti-cancer therapies [15]. Research in human models including a prospective cohort study evaluating whether microbiota composition is correlated with the effectiveness of chemotherapy in colorectal cancer is ongoing [13].

5. Manipulation of the Microbiome as a Component of Cancer Treatment

If the microbiome plays such an important role in the development and treatment of colorectal cancer, does that mean we can alter the microbiome to benefit patients? Current research has approached this question in several different ways (Table 1). Specifically—can manipulating the microbiome be used as a means to help prevent cancer from developing? Can it help prevent or alleviate the adverse effects of therapy for patients who have already been diagnosed? In addition, can it help improve the oncological outcomes such as overall survival?

Table 1. Human studies evaluating probiotics in cancer prevention and treatment.

Study Name	Study Type	Population	Intervention/Cohort Arms	Summary of Key Results
Studies evaluating probiotics and cancer prevention:				
Rafter 2007 [42]	RCT[1]	Colon cancer ($n = 37$) & polypectomized ($n = 43$) patients	SYN1[2] + LCG[3] + BB12[4] vs. placebo	Several CRC[5] biomarkers altered favorably (e.g., decreased genotoxin exposure, IL-2[6], and IFNγ[7])
Ishikawa 2005 [43]	RCT	Tumor-free patients with history of ≥2 colorectal tumors removed ($n = 398$)	Wheat bran vs. *Lactobacillus casei* vs. both vs. neither	No significant difference in colorectal tumor occurrence rate with wheat bran or *L. casei*. However, atypia of tumors was lower in the *L. casei* group.
Pala 2011 [44]	Prospective cohort study	EPIC-Italy cohort ($n = 45,241$)	Yogurt intake by tertile[8]	CRC occurrence was significantly lower in highest vs. lowest tertile of yogurt intake. HR[9] = 0.62 (95% CI[10], 0.46–0.83).
Studies evaluating probiotics and alleviating adverse effects of cancer therapy:				
Mego 2015 [20]	RCT	CRC patients starting treatment with irinotecan-based therapy ($n = 46$)[11]	Colon Dophilus™ probiotic formula vs. placebo	Reduced incidence in probiotic group of severe diarrhea (0% vs. 17.4%, $p = 0.11$) and diarrhea overall (39.1% vs. 60.9%, $p = 0.11$), but not statistically significant.
Osterlund 2007 [45]	RCT	Post-resection CRC patients requiring adjuvant chemotherapy ($n = 150$)	Randomized to 5-FU via Mayo regimen vs. de Gramont regimen, then randomized to LGG vs. no probiotic	Less grade 3–4 diarrhea in patients receiving LGG (22% vs. 37%, $p = 0.027$)
Fuccio 2009 [46]	Meta-analysis	Three RCTs evaluating probiotic supplementation to prevent radiation induced diarrhea ($n = 632$). One RCT evaluating therapeutic role.	Probiotic supplementation vs. placebo/control	No significant difference in rates of radiation-induced diarrhea between probiotic and control arms in preventative trials (OR[12] 0.47, 95% CI 0.13–1.67) or in the single therapeutic trial
Kotzampassi 2015 [21]	RCT	Patients undergoing surgery for CRC ($n = 168$)[13]	Probiotic formulation[14] vs. placebo	Significant decrease in all major post-operative complications in probiotics arm (28.6% vs. 48.8%, $p = 0.010$, OR 0.42)
Krebs 2016 [18]	RCT	Patients undergoing surgery for CRC ($n = 73$)	Preoperative prebiotics[15] vs. preoperative synbiotics[16] vs. mechanical bowel cleansing	No statistical difference in systemic inflammatory response, postoperative course, or complication rate
Studies evaluating probiotics and cancer outcomes:				
Aso 1995 [47]	RCT	Patients with superficial transitional cell carcinoma of the bladder after transurethral resection ($n = 138$)	Oral *L. casei* preparation vs. placebo	Reduced recurrence rate in patients with primary multiple tumors or recurrent single tumors ($p = 0.01$), but not with recurrent multiple tumors
Naito 2008 [48]	RCT	Patients with superficial bladder cancer after transurethral resection and intravesicular epirubicin ($n = 202$)	Intravesicular epirubicin plus *Lactobacillus casei* vs. epirubicin alone	Three-year recurrence-free survival rate was significantly higher in the group receiving *L. casei* (74.6% vs. 59.9%, $p = 0.0234$), no difference in PFS[17] or OS[18]

[1] Randomized control trial. [2] Synbiotic preparation-oligofructose-enriched inulin. [3] *Lactobacillus rhamnosus* GG. [4] *Bifidobacterium lactis* Bb12. [5] Colorectal cancer. [6] Interleukin-2. [7] Interferon gamma. [8] As assessed by a dietary questionnaire. [9] Hazard ratio. [10] Confidence interval. [11] Study prematurely terminated due to slow accrual. [12] Odds ratio. [13] Study prematurely stopped due to efficacy in the primary outcome. [14] Consisting of *Lactobacillus acidophilus*, *L. plantarum*, *Bifidobacterium lactis*, and *Saccharomyces boulardii*. [15] Consisting of betaglucan, inulin, pectin, and resistant starch. [16] Consisting of the prebiotic formulation plus *Pediacoccus pentosaceus* 5-33:3, *Leuconostoc mesenteroides* 32-77:1, *Lactobacillus casei* subspecies *paracasei* 19, and *Lactobacillus plantarum* 2362. [17] Progression free survival. [18] Overall survival.

5.1. Cancer Prevention

There have been a number of studies in both mouse and human models exploring whether manipulation of the microbiome can prevent cancer development. In colorectal cancer specifically, probiotics are reported to have several cancer-preventative mechanisms that have been shown to operate via intraluminal and systemic effects as well as directly on the intestinal mucosa [49]. In these studies, probiotics have been shown to competitively exclude pathogenic intestinal flora [50,51], alter intestinal microflora enzyme activity [52], reduce carcinogenic secondary bile acids [53], bind carcinogens and mutagens, and increase short chain fatty acid production. Probiotics have also been shown to decrease DNA damage [54] at the level of the intestinal mucosa and help maintain an intestinal barrier function [55].

Several studies have looked into the role of probiotics in the prevention of colon cancer and have shown that they appear to have an inhibitory effect on the development of tumors and precancerous lesions even though the effect is not entirely consistent across studies [56]. In one randomized, double-blind, placebo-controlled trial, patients with colon cancer and polypectomized patients were administered a synbiotic consisting of oligofructose-enriched inulin, *Lactobacillus rhamnosus GG*, and *Bifidobacterium lactis Bb12* [57]. Biomarker testing, toxicity assays, and colorectal tissue biopsy samples were checked over the 12-week course of the study with favorable results. Synbiotic administration was associated with reduced colorectal proliferation, reduced capacity of fecal water to induce necrosis in colonic cells, and an improved epithelial barrier function. Colon cancer patients were also noted to have increased production of interferon gamma and assays performed on colon biopsy samples in polypectomized patients showed decreased exposure to genotoxins. Currently, there is very limited human data directly evaluating colorectal cancer risk in relation to specific characteristics or manipulation of the microbiome. A 2005 trial evaluated colorectal tumor recurrence in 398 men and women with a history of removing at least two prior colorectal tumors who were divided into groups receiving a dietary fiber supplement, *Lactobacillus casei*, both, or neither [43]. While there was no significant difference in the development of new colorectal tumors between the groups, the occurrence rate of tumors with moderate or higher-grade atypia was significantly lower in the group receiving *L. casei*. In addition, a large Italian prospective cohort trial showed that self-reported yogurt intake had an inverse association with colorectal cancer risk (HR 0.65 [95% CI, 0.48–0.89] between the highest and lowest tertile) after accounting for potential confounding factors such as BMI, smoking, and physical activity [44]. While these studies are a long way from showing any clinical role for probiotics in colorectal cancer prevention, they suggest that further study may hold promise.

5.2. Alleviating Adverse Effects

Given that previous studies have shown a symptomatic benefit in benign gastrointestinal conditions such as pouchitis and infectious diarrhea, it stands to reason that probiotics may be beneficial in mitigating the adverse gastrointestinal effects of cancer treatment. Mouse studies have supported this hypothesis. For instance, one 2015 study showed that mice treated with intraperitoneally-injected 5-FU developed diarrhea, but their symptoms were improved when given a probiotic suspension. These mice demonstrated the repairing of damage in the jejunal villi as well as reduced mRNA expression of TNF-alpha, IL-1 beta, and IL-6 in intestinal tissue [57]. In another study, mice given with the probiotic mixture VSL#3 had reduced the severity of weight loss and diarrhea after administration of irinotecan as well as reduced apoptosis in the small and large intestine on histological examination [58].

Probiotics also seem to help alleviate non-GI adverse effects as well. A separate study looked at the effect of administering *L. casei* and *L. rhamnosus* strains to mice receiving cyclophosphamide. Mice receiving probiotics demonstrated increased immature myeloid progenitors in bone marrow with early recovery of neutrophils in the peripheral blood, improved phagocytic cell recruitment to infectious sites, and increased resistance to opportunistic infection with *Candida albicans* [59].

There is limited human data evaluating whether probiotics can help improve tolerance to chemotherapy. In one randomized control trial, colorectal cancer patients starting treatment with irinotecan were concurrently given either placebo or a probiotic containing 10 different strains of bacteria. Unfortunately, the trial was discontinued prematurely due to slow accrual with only 46 out of 220 planned patients enrolled. While the study did show a trend toward reduced frequency of severe diarrhea and use of antidiarrheal drugs in the group receiving probiotics, the study was very limited due to its size [20]. A 2007 clinical trial evaluated 150 patients randomly assigned to receive one of two 5-FU-based chemotherapy regimens (Mayo regimen versus simplified de Gramont regimen) and further randomized to receive or not receive *Lactobacillus rhamnosus GG* with fiber as a supplement during chemotherapy [45]. In total, 26% of the patients received pelvic radiation therapy. Patients receiving *Lactobacillus* had a lower incidence of grade 3 or grade 4 diarrhea (22% vs. 37%, $p = 0.027$), less abdominal discomfort, and had fewer hospitalizations and chemotherapy dose reductions due to bowel toxicity. However, the study was limited due to lack of blinding and placebo control.

Probiotics have also been studied in the setting of radiation therapy and surgery for the treatment of cancer. In a 2009 meta-analysis of four studies evaluating probiotics in the treatment of radiation enteritis, some of the individual studies showed a significant effect, but the meta-analysis did not demonstrate an overall benefit when all trials were taken into account [46]. Nevertheless, research has shown that intestinal bacteria contribute to radiation-induced injury and repair [60]. Given the variation of probiotic strains and doses between studies, it would be premature to rule out probiotics as a possible treatment in the current state of research.

Results have been mixed in trials evaluating probiotics as an adjunctive treatment to surgery as well. In one study of 168 patients evaluated after colorectal surgery for cancer, those receiving a four-probiotic regimen had a significantly decreased rate of all postoperative major complications when compared to the placebo arm (28.6% vs. 48.8%, $p = 0.010$) [21]. However, a separate randomized trial evaluating 73 patients who received a prebiotic, a synbiotic, or a standard bowel prep prior to resection for colorectal cancer found no difference in the systemic inflammatory marker response and no effect on post-operative course or complication rates [18].

5.3. Cancer Outcomes

Data evaluating probiotics as a potential means to prevent cancer or to alleviate the adverse effects of cancer treatment is limited, but data evaluating whether probiotics affect cancer treatment outcomes is even scarcer. Currently, there does not appear to be any published randomized control trials in the literature evaluating whether manipulation of microbiota in patients receiving treatment for colorectal cancer can affect outcomes such as the objective response rate or progression-free survival. Two randomized control trials, however, did evaluate the effect of probiotics on cancer outcomes in bladder cancer. The first, which is a 1995 trial, evaluated 138 patients with primary bladder tumors treated with transurethral resection of the bladder tumor (TURBT). Afterwards, the patients were treated with either an oral preparation of *Lactobacillus casei* or placebo. Patients receiving probiotics had a significant decrease in cancer recurrence with a corrected cumulative recurrence-free rate at one year of 79.2% versus 54.9% with placebo ($p = 0.01$) [59]. A later trial in 2008 evaluated 207 patients with superficial bladder cancer. Patients were treated with TURBT followed by transurethral epirubicin with one group of 100 patients receiving an oral *Lactobacillus casei* preparation once daily for one year. Three-year recurrence free survival was significantly higher in the group receiving probiotics (74.6% vs. 59.9%, $p = 0.02$). However, overall survival did not differ between the two groups [48]. While it is difficult to draw generalized conclusions from these trials, they do suggest that further clinical study would be reasonable especially given the relative safety [61] of administering probiotics.

6. Discussion

We currently have only a very primitive understanding of the microbiome and how it functions in the human body. There is an ongoing debate over even the fundamentals of the microbiome. We know that it is vital to human health, but we are far from being able to define what a "healthy" human microbiome looks like. We know that certain functions such as regulation of the immune system and gut mucosal barrier are beneficial, but it stands to reason that there are a vast number of critical microbiome functions that have not yet been discovered.

Luckily, we do not need a perfect understanding before translating knowledge of the microbiome into clinical interventions. Studies so far have suggested that restoring function to the microbiome can have beneficial effects in the prevention of cancer and in improving the effectiveness and safety of cancer treatment. As we have seen, administration of certain *Lactobacillus* and *Bifidobacterium* strains is associated with biochemical and histologic changes that may decrease the risk of developing malignancy [50,51]. Other *Lactobacillus* [40], *Bifidobacterium* [17], and *Bacteroides* [16] strains seem to play critical roles in the effectiveness of certain cytotoxic and immune therapies. Nonetheless, the bulk of research in these topics has been in animal models. Data from human research, particularly in clinical trials evaluating whether probiotics or synbiotics can alleviate the adverse effects of various cancer therapies, has so far shown mixed results.

These mixed results are not necessarily unexpected given the early state of clinical research into probiotics, colorectal cancer, and the microbiome. Colorectal cancer provides many different populations, cancer treatment modalities, and patient outcomes to study, which means a probiotic regimen showing a benefit in one cohort will not necessarily show a benefit in all colorectal cancer patients. Several of the clinical trials evaluating probiotics in cancer patients suffer from major limitations ranging from lack of blinding and a placebo control group [56] to inadequate patient accrual [20]. While some of these studies suggest that probiotic therapy is helpful, it will take further clinical research with larger, more diverse patient populations to determine if there is true benefit.

In addition, while some individual probiotic formulations have been studied across multiple clinical trials, there is no strong evidence favoring one formulation over another. Certain bacterial species seem to provide specific helpful functions, but translating this knowledge into clinically beneficial therapies will likely prove difficult. For instance, as previously noted in mouse studies, commensal *Bifidobacterium* seems to be important in the effectiveness of anti-PD-L1 therapy [17]. If this were experimentally proven in humans as well, many questions would remain. Would we be able to overcome a *Bifidobacterium* "deficiency" through the administration of oral probiotics or synbiotics? If so, is there a minimum dosage in colony forming units (CFUs) that would need to be administered for the treatment to be effective? Could other, non-*Bifidobacterium* strains of commensal bacteria perform equivalent functions that amplify the effectiveness of anti-PD-L1 treatments?

Additionally, what is the benefit, if any, of administering multiple strains of probiotics in a single formulation? There are innumerable interactions between individual bacterial strains in the gut microbiota and certain microbiome compositions appear to make individuals more or less susceptible to colonization with certain pathogenic bacteria [62]. It stands to reason that multiple types of bacteria with anti-tumor effects may synergize when administered together. In fact, many of the clinical trials reviewed in this article examined probiotic formulations instead of probiotics consisting of a single strain. Presumably using probiotic strains with different beneficial mechanisms of action may elicit a better outcome than any one alone and there may be other mechanisms by which commensal bacteria cooperate with each other. However, it is also entirely possible that the opposite is true and giving certain probiotics in combination will cause them to limit each other's effectiveness.

Ultimately, in order to realize the promise of microbiome-related therapies, research will need to focus on developing defined probiotic therapy regimens with specific strains and doses that may result in a reproducible clinical benefit. Even then, we will need additional research to determine whether a synergistic effect between probiotics and anti-cancer drugs will translate into improved oncologic outcomes such as progression-free or overall survival.

7. Conclusions

Studies evaluating the gut microbiome have shown promising connections between it and the pathogenesis and treatment of colorectal cancer. Further translational research and clinical trials in human subjects are warranted to investigate the possibility of manipulating the microbiome to improve outcomes in colorectal cancer.

Funding: This research received no external funding.

Conflicts of Interest: The authors declare no conflict of interest.

References

1. Torre, L.A.; Bray, F.; Siegel, R.L.; Ferlay, J.; Lortet-Tieulent, J.; Jemal DVM, A. Global cancer statistics, 2012. *Cancer J. Clin.* **2015**, *65*, 87–108. [CrossRef] [PubMed]
2. Siegel, R.L.; Miller, K.D.; Jemal, A. Cancer Statistics, 2017. *Cancer J. Clin.* **2017**, *67*, 7–30. [CrossRef] [PubMed]
3. Jemal, A.; Ward, E.M.; Johnson, C.J.; Cronin, K.A.; Ma, J.; Ryerson, A.B.; Mariotto, A.; Lake, A.J.; Wilson, R.; Sherman, R.L.; et al. Annual Report to the Nation on the Status of Cancer, 1975–2014, Featuring Survival. *J. Natl. Cancer Inst.* **2017**, *109*. [CrossRef] [PubMed]
4. Edge, S.B.; Byrd, D.R.; Compton, C.C.; Frita, A.G.; Greene, F.L.; Trotti, A. Colon and Rectum. In *Cuccurullo, V. AJCC Cancer Staging Handbook: From the AJCC Cancer Staging Manual*, 7th ed.; Cuccurullo, V., Mansi, L., Eds.; Springer: New York, NY, USA, 2010; p. 143.
5. Ursell, L.K.; Metcalf, J.L.; Parfrey, L.W.; Knight, R. Defining the human microbiome. *Nutr. Rev.* **2012**, *70*, S38–S44. [CrossRef] [PubMed]
6. The NIH HMP Working Group; Peterson, J.; Garges, S.; Giovanni, M.; McInnes, P.; Wang, L.; Schloss, J.A.; Bonazzi, V.; McEwen, J.E.; Wetterstrand, K.A.; et al. The NIH human microbiome project. *Genome Res.* **2009**, *19*, 2317–2323. [CrossRef] [PubMed]
7. Qin, J.; Li, R.; Raes, J.; Arumugam, M.; Burgdorf, K.S.; Manichanh, C.; Nielsen, T.; Pons, F.; Levenez, F.; Yamada, T.; et al. A human gut microbial gene catalogue established by metagenomic sequencing. *Nature* **2010**, *464*, 59–65. [CrossRef] [PubMed]
8. Lloyd-Price, J.; Abu-Ali, G.; Huttenhower, C. The healthy human microbiome. *Genome Med.* **2016**, *8*, 51. [CrossRef] [PubMed]
9. Barlow, G.M.; Yu, A.; Mathur, R. Role of the Gut Microbiome in Obesity and Diabetes Mellitus. *Nutr. Clin. Pract.* **2015**, *30*, 787–797. [CrossRef] [PubMed]
10. Ambalam, P.; Raman, M.; Purama, R.K.; Doble, M. Probiotics, prebiotics and colorectal cancer prevention. *Best Pract. Res. Clin. Gastroenterol.* **2016**, *30*, 119–131. [CrossRef] [PubMed]
11. Zackular, J.P.; Baxter, N.T.; Iverson, K.D.; Iverson, K.D.; Sadler, W.D.; Petrosino, J.F.; Chen, G.Y.; Schloss, P.D. The gut microbiome modulates colon tumorigenesis. *mBio* **2013**, *4*, e000692-13. [CrossRef] [PubMed]
12. Raskov, H.; Burcharth, J.; Pommergaard, H.C. Linking Gut Microbiota to Colorectal Cancer. *J. Cancer* **2017**, *8*, 3378–3395. [CrossRef] [PubMed]
13. Aarnoutse, R.; De Vos-Geelen, J.M.P.G.M.; Penders, J.; Boerma, E.G.; Warmerdam, F.A.R.M.; Goorts, B.; Olde Damink, S.W.M.; Soons, Z.; Rensen, S.S.M.; Smidt, M.L. Study protocol on the role of intestinal microbiota in colorectal cancer treatment: A pathway to personalized medicine 2.0. *Int. J. Colorectal. Dis.* **2017**, *32*, 1077–1084. [CrossRef] [PubMed]
14. Iida, N.; Dzutsev, A.; Stewart, C.A.; Smith, L.; Bouladoux, N.; Weingarten, R.A.; Molina, D.A.; Salcedo, R.; Back, T.; Cramer, T.; et al. Commensal bacteria control cancer response to therapy modulating the tumor microenvironment. *Science* **2013**, *342*, 967–970. [CrossRef] [PubMed]
15. Pennisi, E. Biomedicine. Cancer therapies use a little help from microbial friends. *Science* **2013**, *342*, 921. [CrossRef] [PubMed]
16. Vetizou, M.; Pitt, J.M.; Dalliere, R.; Lepage, P.; Waldschmitt, N.; Flament, C.; Rusakiewicz, S.; Routy, B.; Roberti, M.P.; Duong, C.P.M.; et al. Anticancer immunotherapy by CTLA-4 blockade relies on the gut microbiota. *Science* **2015**, *350*. [CrossRef] [PubMed]
17. Sivan, A.; Corrales, L.; Hubert, N. Commensal Bifidobacterium promotes antitumor immunity and facilitates anti-PD-L1 efficacy. *Science* **2015**, *350*, 1084–1089. [CrossRef] [PubMed]

18. Krebs, B. Prebiotic and synbiotic treatment before colorectal surgery–randomised double blind trial. *Coll. Antropol.* **2016**, *40*, 35–40. [PubMed]
19. Della, P.; Sansotta, G.; Donato, V.; Frosina, P.; Messina, G.; De Renzis, C.; Famularo, G. Use of probiotics for prevention of radiation-induced diarrhea. *World J. Gastroenterol.* **2007**, *13*, 912–915. [CrossRef]
20. Mego, M.; Chovanec, J.; Vochyanova-Andrezalova, I.; Konkolovsky, P.; Mikulova, M.; Reckova, M.; Miskovska, V.; Bysticky, B.; Beniak, J.; Medvecova, L.; et al. Prevention of irinotecan induced diarrhea by probiotics: A randomized double blind, placebo controlled pilot study. *Complement. Ther. Med.* **2015**, *23*, 356–362. [CrossRef] [PubMed]
21. Kotzampassi, K.; Stavrou, G.; Damoraki, G.; Georgitsi, M.; Basdanis, G.; Tsaousi, G.; Giamarellos-Bourboulis, E.J. A four-probiotics regimen reduces postoperative complications after colorectal surgery: A randomized, double-blind, placebo-controlled study. *World J. Surg.* **2015**, *39*, 2776–2783. [CrossRef] [PubMed]
22. Turnbaugh, P.J.; Ridaura, V.K.; Faith, J.J.; Turnbaugh, P.J.; Knight, R.; Gorfon, J.I. The effect of diet on the human gut microbiome: A metagenomic analysis in humanized gnotobiotic mice. *Sci. Transl. Med.* **2009**, *11*. [CrossRef] [PubMed]
23. Wasilewski, A.; Zielinska, M.; Storr, M.; Fichna, J. Beneficial effects of probiotics, prebiotics, synbiotics, and psychobiotics in inflammatory bowel disease. *Inflamm. Bowel Dis.* **2015**, *21*, 1674–1682. [CrossRef] [PubMed]
24. Gibson, G.R.; Beatty, E.R.; Wang, X.; Cummings, J.H. Selective stimulation of bifidobacteria in the human colon by oligofructose and inulin. *Gastroenterology* **1995**, *108*, 975–982. [CrossRef]
25. Looijer-van Langen, M.A.C.; Dieleman, L.A. Prebiotics in chronic intestinal inflammation. *Inflamm. Bowel Dis.* **2009**, *15*, 454–462. [CrossRef] [PubMed]
26. Vanderpool, C.; Yan, F.; Polk, D.B. Mechanisms of probiotic action: Implications for therapeutic applications in inflammatory bowel disease. *Inflamm. Bowel Dis.* **2008**, *14*, 1585. [CrossRef] [PubMed]
27. Holubar, S.D.; Cima, R.R.; Sandborn, W.J.; Pardi, D.S. Treatment and prevention of pouchitis after ileal pouch-anal anastomosis for chronic ulcerative colitis. *Cochrane Database Syst. Rev.* **2010**, *6*. [CrossRef]
28. Allen, S.J.; Martinez, E.G.; Gregorio, G.V.; Dans, L.F. Probiotics for treating acute infectious diarrhoea. *Cochrane Database Syst. Rev.* **2010**, *2010*. [CrossRef] [PubMed]
29. Van Niel, C.W.; Feudtner, C.; Garrison, M.M.; Christakis, D.A. Lactobacillus therapy for acute infectious diarrhea in children: A meta-analysis. *Pediatrics* **2002**, *109*, 678–684. [CrossRef] [PubMed]
30. Dimidi, E.; Christodoulides, S.; Fragkos, K.C.; Scott, S.M.; Whelan, K. The effect of probiotics on functional constipation in adults: A systematic review and meta-analysis of randomized control trials. *Am. J. Clin. Nutr.* **2014**, *100*, 1075–1084. [CrossRef] [PubMed]
31. Kasai, C.; Sugimoto, K.; Moritani, I.; Tanaka, J.; Oya, Y.; Inoue, H.; Tamede, M.; Shiraki, K.; Ito, M.; Takei, Y.; et al. Comparison of human gut microbiota in control subjects and patients with colorectal carcinoma in adenoma: Terminal restriction fragment length polymorphism and next-generation sequencing analyses. *Oncol. Rep.* **2016**, *35*, 325–333. [CrossRef] [PubMed]
32. Flemer, B.; Lynch, D.B.; Brown, J.M.R.; Jeffery, I.B.; Ryan, F.J.; Claesson, M.J.; O'Riordain, M.; Shanahan, F.; O'Toole, P.W. Tumour-associated and non-tumour-associated microbiota in colorectal cancer. *Gut* **2016**, *66*, 633–643. [CrossRef] [PubMed]
33. Klampfer, L. Cytokines, inflammation and colon cancer. *Curr. Cancer Drug Targets* **2011**, *11*, 451–464. [CrossRef] [PubMed]
34. Li, S.; Konstantinov, S.R.; Smits, R.; Peppelenbosch, M.P. Bacterial biofilms in colorectal cancer initiation and progression. *Trends Mol. Med.* **2017**, *23*, 18–30. [CrossRef] [PubMed]
35. Wu, S.; Rhee, K.-J.; Albesiano, E.; Rabizadeh, S.; Wu, X.; Yen, H.-R.; Huso, D.L.; Brancati, F.L.; Wick, E.; McAllister, F.; et al. A human colonic commensal promotes tumorigenesis via activation of T helper type 17 T cell responses. *Nat. Med.* **2009**, *15*, 1016–1022. [CrossRef] [PubMed]
36. Kostik, A.D.; Gevers, D.; Pedamallu, C.S.; Michaud, M.; Duke, F.; Earl, A.M.; Ojesina, A.I.; Jung, J.; Bass, A.J.; Tabernero, J.; et al. Genomic analysis identified association of Fusobacterium with colorectal carcinoma. *Genome Res.* **2012**, *22*, 292–298. [CrossRef] [PubMed]
37. Castellarin, M.; Warren, R.L.; Freeman, J.D.; Dreolini, L.; Krzywinki, M.; Strauss, J.; Barnes, R.; Watson, R.; Allen-Vercoe, E.; Moore, R.A.; et al. Fusobacterium nucleatum infection is prevalent in human colorectal carcinoma. *Genome Res.* **2012**, *22*, 299–306. [CrossRef] [PubMed]

38. Shang, F.; Liu, H. Fusobacterium nucleatum and colorectal cancer: A review. *World J. Gastrointest. Oncol.* **2018**, *10*, 71–81. [CrossRef] [PubMed]
39. Ericcson, A.C.; Akter, S.; Hanson, M.M.; Busi, S.B.; Parker, T.W.; Schehr, R.J.; Hankins, M.A.; Ahner, C.E.; Davis, J.W.; Franklin, C.L.; et al. Differential susceptibility to colorectal cancer due to naturally occurring gut microbiota. *Oncotarget* **2015**, *6*, 33689–33704. [CrossRef] [PubMed]
40. An, J.; Ha, E.M. Combination therapy of Lactobacillus plantarum Supernatant and 5-Fluouracil Increases Chemosensitivity in Colorectal Cancer Cells. *J. Microbiol. Biotechnol.* **2016**, *26*, 1490–1503. [CrossRef] [PubMed]
41. Viaud, S.; Saccheri, F.; Mignot, G.; Yamazaki, T.; Daillere, R.; Hannani, D.; Enot, D.P.; Pfirschke, C.; Engblom, C.; Pittet, M.J.; et al. The intestinal microbiota modulates the anticancer immune effects of cyclophosphamide. *Science* **2013**, *342*, 971–976. [CrossRef] [PubMed]
42. Rafter, J.; Bennett, M.; Caderni, G.; Clune, Y.; Hughes, R.; Karlsson, P.C.; Klinder, A.; O'Riordan, M.; O'Sullivan, G.C.; Pool-Zobel, P.; et al. Dietary synbiotics reduce cancer risk factors in polypectomized and colon cancer patients. *Am. J. Clin. Nutr.* **2007**, *85*, 488–496. [CrossRef] [PubMed]
43. Ishikawa, H.; Akedo, I.; Otani, T.; Suzuki, T.; Nakamura, T.; Takeyama, I.; Ishiguro, S.; Miyaoka, E.; Sobue, T.; Kakizoe, T. Randomized trial of dietary fiber and *Lactobacillus casei* administration for prevention of colorectal tumors. *Int. J. Cancer* **2005**, *116*, 752–757. [CrossRef] [PubMed]
44. Pala, V.; Sieri, S.; Berrino, F.; Vineis, P.; Sacerdote, C.; Palli, D.; Masala, G.; Panico, S.; Mattiello, A.; Tumino, R.; et al. Yogurt consumption and risk of colorectal cancer in the Italian European prospective investigation into cancer and nutrition cohort. *Int. J. Cancer* **2011**, *129*, 2712–2719. [CrossRef] [PubMed]
45. Osterlund, P.; Ruotsalainen, T.; Korpela, R.; Ollus, M.; Valta, P.; Kouri, M.; Elomaa, I.; Joensuu, H. Lactobacillus supplementation for diarrhoea related to chemotherapy of colorectal cancer: A randomised study. *Br. J. Cancer* **2007**, *97*, 1028–1034. [CrossRef] [PubMed]
46. Fuccio, L.; Guido, A.; Eusebi, L.H.; Laterza, L.; Grilli, D.; Cennamo, V.; Ceroni, L.; Barbieri, E.; Bazzoil, F. Effects of probiotics for the prevention and treatment of radiation-induced diarrhea. *J. Clin. Gastroenterol.* **2009**, *43*, 506–513. [CrossRef] [PubMed]
47. Aso, Y.; Akaza, H.; Kotake, T.; Tsukamoto, T.; Imai, K.; Naito, S. The BLP Study Group. Preventive effect of a *Lactobacillus casei* preparation on the recurrence of superficial bladder cancer in a double-blind trial. *Eur. Urol.* **1995**, *27*, 104–109. [CrossRef] [PubMed]
48. Naito, S.; Koga, H.; Yamaguchi, A.; Fujimoto, N.; Hasui, Y.; Kuramoto, H.; Iguch, A. Kyushu University Urological Oncology Group. Prevention of recurrence with epirubicin and Lactobacillus casei after transurethral resection of bladder cancer. *J. Urol.* **2008**, *179*, 485–490. [CrossRef] [PubMed]
49. Chong, E.S.L. A potential role of probiotics in colorectal cancer prevention: Review of possible mechanisms of action. *World J. Microbiol. Biotechnol.* **2014**, *30*, 351–374. [CrossRef] [PubMed]
50. Fooks, L.J.; Gibson, G.R. Probiotics as moderators of gut flora. *Br. J. Nutr.* **2002**, *88*, S39–S49. [CrossRef] [PubMed]
51. Tareb, R.; Bernardeau, M.; Geuguen, M.; Vernoux, J.-P. In vitro characterization of aggregation and adhesion properties of viable and heat-killed forms of two probiotic *Lactobacillus* strains and interaction with foodborne zoonotic bacteria, especially *Campylobacter jejuni*. *J. Med. Microbiol.* **2013**, *62*, 637–649. [CrossRef] [PubMed]
52. Verma, A.; Shukla, G. Probiotics *Lacobacillus rhamnosus* GG, Lactobacillus acidophilus suppressed DMH-induced procarcinogenic fecal enzymes and preneoplastic aberrant crypt foci in early colon carcinogenesis in Sprague Dawley rats. *Nutr. Cancer* **2013**, *65*, 84–91. [CrossRef] [PubMed]
53. Sato, S.; Nagai, H.; Igarashi, Y. Effect of probiotics on serum bile acids in patients with ulcerative colitis. *Hepatogastroenterology* **2012**, *59*, 1804–1808. [CrossRef] [PubMed]
54. Oberreuther-Moschner, D.L.; Jahreis, G.; Rechkemmer, G.; Pool-Zobel, B.L. Dietary intervention with the probiotics *Lactobacillus acidophilus* 145 and *Bifidobacterium longum* 913 modulates the potential of human faecal water to induce damage in HT29clone19A cells. *Br. J. Nutr.* **2004**, *91*, 925–932. [CrossRef] [PubMed]
55. Mennigen, R.; Nolte, K.; Rijcken, E.; Utech, M.; Loeffler, B.; Senninger, N.; Bruewer, M. Probiotic mixture VSL#3 protects the epithelial barrier by maintaining tight junction protein expression and preventing apoptosis in a murine model of colitis. *Am. J. Physiol. Gastrointest. Liver Physiol.* **2009**, *296*, G1140–G1149. [CrossRef] [PubMed]
56. Brady, L.J.; Gallaher, D.D.; Busta, F.F. The role of probiotic cultures in the prevention of colon cancer. *J. Nutr.* **2000**, *130*, 410S–414S. [CrossRef] [PubMed]

57. Yeung, C.-Y.; Chan, W.-T.; Jiang, C.-B.; Cheng, M.-L.; Liu, C.-Y.; Chiau, J.-S.C.; Lee, H.-C. Amelioration of chemotherapy-induced intestinal mucositis by orally administered probiotics in a mouse model. *PLoS ONE* **2015**, *10*, e0141402. [CrossRef] [PubMed]
58. Bowen, J.M.; Stringer, A.M.; Gibson, R.J.; Yeoh, A.S.J.; Hannam, S.; Keefe, D.M.K. VSL#3 probiotic treatment reduces chemotherapy-induced diarrhea and weight loss. *Cancer Biol. Ther.* **2007**, *6*, 1449–1454. [PubMed]
59. Salva, S.; Marranzino, G.; Villena, J. Probiotic *Lactobacillus* strains protect against myelosuppression and immunosuppression in cyclophosphamide-treated mice. *Int. Immunopharmacol.* **2014**, *22*, 209–221. [CrossRef] [PubMed]
60. Packey, C.D.; Ciorba, M.A. Microbial influences on the small intestinal response to radiation injury. *Curr. Opin. Gastroenterol.* **2010**, *26*, 88–94. [CrossRef] [PubMed]
61. Redman, M.G.; Ward, E.J.; Phillips, R.S. The efficacy and safety of probiotics in people with cancer: A systematic review. *Ann. Oncol.* **2014**, *25*, 1919–1929. [CrossRef] [PubMed]
62. Baumler, A.J.; Sperandio, V. Interactions between the microbiota and pathogenic bacteria in the gut. *Nature* **2016**, *535*, 85–93. [CrossRef] [PubMed]

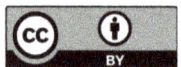

© 2018 by the authors. Licensee MDPI, Basel, Switzerland. This article is an open access article distributed under the terms and conditions of the Creative Commons Attribution (CC BY) license (http://creativecommons.org/licenses/by/4.0/).

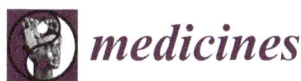

Review

Anticancer Effects of Green Tea and the Underlying Molecular Mechanisms in Bladder Cancer

Yasuyoshi Miyata *, Tomohiro Matsuo, Kyohei Araki, Yuichiro Nakamura, Yuji Sagara, Kojiro Ohba and Hideki Sakai

Department of Urology, Nagasaki University Graduate School of Biomedical Sciences, Nagasaki 852-8501, Japan; tomozo1228@hotmail.com (T.M.); k-araki205@cameo.plala.or.jp (K.A.); yn1238056@yahoo.co.jp (Y.N.); gaasara3@gmail.com (Y.S.); ohba-k@nagasaki-u.ac.jp (K.O.); hsakai@nagasaki-u.ac.jp (H.S.)
* Correspondence: int.doc.miya@m3.dion.ne.jp; Tel.: +81 95-819-7340

Received: 9 July 2018; Accepted: 7 August 2018; Published: 10 August 2018

Abstract: Green tea and green tea polyphenols (GTPs) are reported to inhibit carcinogenesis and malignant behavior in several diseases. Various in vivo and in vitro studies have shown that GTPs suppress the incidence and development of bladder cancer. However, at present, opinions concerning the anticancer effects and preventive role of green tea are conflicting. In addition, the detailed molecular mechanisms underlying the anticancer effects of green tea in bladder cancer remain unclear, as these effects are regulated by several cancer-related factors. A detailed understanding of the pathological roles and regulatory mechanisms at the molecular level is necessary for advancing treatment strategies based on green tea consumption for patients with bladder cancer. In this review, we discuss the anticancer effects of GTPs on the basis of data presented in in vitro studies in bladder cancer cell lines and in vivo studies using animal models, as well as new treatment strategies for patients with bladder cancer, based on green tea consumption. Finally, on the basis of the accumulated data and the main findings, we discuss the potential usefulness of green tea as an antibladder cancer agent and the future direction of green tea-based treatment strategies for these patients.

Keywords: animal model; treatment; bladder cancer; epidemiology; green tea

1. Introduction

Green tea is obtained from the leaves of the plant *Camellia sinensis*, and it is one of the most popular beverages worldwide, particularly in Asia. Green tea is recognized to have health-promoting effects that are attributed to green tea polyphenols (GTPs), such as epicatechin, epigallocatechin, epicatechin-3-gallate (ECG), and epigallocatechin-3-gallate (EGCG) [1]. In addition, its antioxidant, anti-inflammatory, and antibacterial properties have been reported to provide various benefits to its consumers [2]. Several investigators have reported that the addition of GTPs to drinking water can prevent carcinogenesis and the development of various types of malignancies [3–5]. In addition, laboratory-based evidence of the anticancer effects of GTPs has been increasing [4,6]. On the other hand, other studies have shown that green tea consumption does not decrease the risk for various types of cancers, including brain cancer and breast cancer [7,8]. In addition, a meta-analysis of published case-control and cohort studies showed that green tea consumption is not associated with risk of pancreatic cancer [9]. Furthermore, no significant association between green tea consumption and colon cancer risk was observed (summary RR: 0.99; 95% CI: 0.79, 1.24) in prospective cohort studies [10]. Additionally, it has been reported that green tea consumption might be associated with an increased risk of upper aerodigestive tract cancer [11]. Taken together, the anticancer effects of green tea consumption and GTPs remain controversial. With regard to bladder cancer, various in vivo and in vitro studies have provided inconsistent results.

Below, we first present a general discussion on the relationship between green tea consumption and cancer risk on the basis of data from epidemiological studies, the mechanisms underlying these anticancer effects, the safety and adverse effects of GTPs, and trials of treatment strategies based on green tea consumption. Then, we present a detailed review of these topics with a focus on bladder cancer. Previously, excellent reviews of studies, particularly epidemiological investigations, on the relationship between green tea consumption and bladder cancer risk have been published [12,13]. Therefore, in the present review, we paid attention to the molecular mechanisms underlying the anticancer effects, findings from studies involving animal models, and novel treatment strategies based on green tea consumption for patients with bladder cancer, as these topics have been less well addressed in previous reviews.

2. Anticancer Effects of Green Tea Polyphenols

GTPs exhibit anticancer effects via the regulation of different cancer-related processes and factors, including DNA methylation, histone modification, micro-RNA, and proteins [5,14–17]. They also play an important role via the regulation of apoptosis, growth, invasion, and angiogenesis in various types of malignancies [13,15,18,19]. A recent study showed that GTPs can influence the pathological roles of not only cancer cells, but also cancer stem cells [17]. These findings have led to a hypothesis that GTPs have strong anticancer effects in vivo and in vitro. In the next section, findings that support this hypothesis are discussed.

2.1. Anticancer Effects Shown in Epidemiological Studies

When discussing the anticancer effects of GTPs, it is necessary to focus on the different phases in the natural evolution of malignant cells. Briefly, green tea extracts are thought to be useful for primary prevention (prevention and delay of cancer onset) and tertiary prevention (prevention of recurrence and metastasis) [17]. With regard to primary prevention, several epidemiological studies have shown that the average age at cancer onset in individuals with high levels of green tea consumption was significantly higher than that in individuals with low levels of green tea consumption [17,20,21]. These studies have also shown that the consumption of more than 10 cups of green tea was associated with a reduced incidence of lung, colorectum, liver, and stomach cancer [17,20,21]. Furthermore, several reports have shown that GTPs were effective in preventing transformation from a premalignant status to frank malignancy [14,22].

With regard to tertiary cancer prevention, on the other hand, one study reported that the recurrence rate for stage I and stage II breast cancer was significantly lower for patients consuming $\geq$5 cups of green tea daily (16.7%) than in those consuming $\leq$4 cups (24.3%; $p < 0.005$) [23]. However, these preventive effects were not observed for stage III breast cancer recurrence. Another report stated that the hazard ratio for stage I breast cancer recurrence showed a statistically significant decrease (hazard ratio, 0.43; 95% confidential interval, 0.22–0.84) [24]. Similar preventive effects on cancer recurrence have also been reported for other cancers. For example, a study showed that the recurrence rate for colorectal cancer was significantly lower in an experimental group (daily consumption of green tea plus tablets of green tea extracts (GTEs) than in a control group (31.0% vs. 15.0%; $p < 0.05$) [25]. In addition, GTEs reportedly showed inhibitory effects on metastasis in various types of malignancies. For example, lung metastasis from melanoma was inhibited by GTEs in an animal experiment [26].

2.2. Mechanisms Underlying the Anticancer Effects of Green Tea

Various cancer-related molecules have been reported to be modulated by GTPs. In fact, many studies have reported that GTPs inhibited cell growth and induced apoptosis in various types of malignancies [19,27,28]. In addition, these polyphenols modulate the functions of various cancer-related signaling molecules. For example, the function and expression of vascular endothelial growth factor (VEGF), which is a strong stimulator of angiogenesis, are mediated by GTPs in oral cancer and esophageal squamous cell carcinoma [14,29]. Furthermore, in these malignancies, cyclin

D1, which is a cell cycle regulator, and caspase-3, which is an important determinant for apoptosis, are associated with GTPs [14,29].

EGCG has also been reported to affect the pathological behavior of stem cells in several cancers. For example, they inhibited the proliferation and induced the apoptosis of lung cancer stem cells [30] and suppressed tumor spheroid formation by colorectal cancer stem cells [16].

Numerous previous reports have presented detailed information on the mechanisms underlying the general anticancer effects of green tea; thus, we present the details only for bladder cancer.

2.3. Cancer Treatment Strategies Based on Green Tea Consumption

While GTPs inhibit tumor growth in human lung cancer cell lines, their inhibitory effects were approximately 250-fold less effective than those of doxorubicin (Adriamycin) [31]. Therefore, it has been suggested that GTPs are more suitable for use in cancer prevention than as cancer treatment [17]. In fact, chemoprevention by oral administration of green tea catechins was investigated in volunteers with high-grade prostate intraepithelial neoplasia, a precancerous change [22]. Furthermore, EGCG administration was reported to be useful as an adjuvant therapy after complete tumor resection [32]. Various GTPs can also increase the sensitivity of anticancer agents and prevent drug resistance [33,34]. In fact, new cancer treatment strategies using a combination of GTPs and anticancer agents, such as cisplatin, paclitaxel, and tamoxifen, have been recommended for several types of malignancies [35,36]. The molecular mechanisms underlying these synergistic effects are partially clear. For example, in osteosarcoma, SOX overlapping transcript variant 7 is known to contribute to an improvement in the clinical efficacy of combination therapy with EGCG and doxorubicin via inhibition of both autophagy and stemness [37]. In addition to anticancer agents, various natural compounds have also been shown to exhibit anticancer effects when combined with GTPs. For example, in a xenograft model of human leukemia, the oral intake of green tea and intraperitoneal injection of quercetin, which is a polyphenol present in fruits and vegetables, induced apoptosis and suppressed tumor growth [38]. Furthermore, another study reported that EGCG and quercetin enhanced the anticancer effects of doxorubicin via regulation of cell cycle arrest and apoptosis in prostate cancer [39].

As mentioned above, the anticancer effects of GTPs are relatively weak, and a higher concentration of GTPs near cancer cells is considered to improve their anticancer effects. Polymeric micelles are used as the drug-delivery systems in various treatments. In recent years, several anticancer drug-loaded micellar nanocomplexes based on GTE-derivatives have been developed [40,41]. A micellar nanocomplex based on the self-assembly of EGCG and doxorubicin inhibited tumor growth in a xenograft model of human liver cancer [41]; similar results were reported for a micellar nanocomplex prepared by complexation of oligomerized EGCG with trastuzumab (Herceptin) in a mouse model of breast cancer [40]. These findings indicate that more detailed in vivo studies and clinical trials of such combined therapies are important for development of new treatment strategies of bladder cancer.

3. Bladder Cancer and Green Tea

Bladder cancer is a common malignancy in 43 countries around the globe, although the incidence among men, women, and both sexes has decreased in 11, 10, and 12 countries, respectively [42]. Bladder cancer imposes a substantial psychological, physical, and economic burden, and its prognosis is poor, despite various multidisciplinary therapeutic approaches, particularly in cases with muscle invasion and/or metastasis [43]. Therefore, more detailed information will be useful for devising preventive and treatment strategies.

Many studies have focused on the clinical benefits of food choices in terms of chemoprevention, treatment, and survival in bladder cancer [44]. Furthermore, complementary and alternative medicine (CAM), defined as a diverse medical and healthcare system, is recognized as a strategy commonly used by patients with malignancies, including bladder cancer [45]. Green tea consumption and GTPs intake are suggested as CAM strategies [46].

3.1. Epidemiological Studies on Bladder Cancer

3.1.1. Case-Control and Cohort Studies

As mentioned above, no consensus has been derived from the findings of epidemiological studies on green tea consumption, and the effects thereof on carcinogenesis and tumor development and growth remain controversial. Similarly, with regard to bladder cancer, opinions about the relationship between green tea consumption and cancer risk are conflicting. For example, it was reported that the risk of bladder cancer in individuals with high green tea consumption (≥ 0.14 servings/day) was lower than that in individuals who never consumed the beverage (odds ratio, 0.60; 95% confidential interval, 0.45–0.79; $p < 0.001$) [47]. However, to our knowledge, this is the only study supporting the hypothesis that a high level of green tea consumption suppresses the risk of bladder cancer. On the other hand, surprisingly, another study reported that the risk of bladder cancer was significantly higher for individuals who consumed five to nine cups of green tea daily than in those who did not consume green tea (odds ratio, 2.67; 95% confidential interval, 0.49–2.84) [48]. However, the same study also showed that bladder cancer risk was similar for individuals who consumed ≥ 10 cups daily than for those who did not consume green tea (odds ratio, 1.18; 95% confidential interval, 1.44–4.94) [48]. Table 1 summarizes the findings of previous studies on the relationship between green tea consumption and bladder cancer risk.

Table 1. Previous reports on the relationship between green tea consumption and bladder cancer risk.

Case-Control Study				Cohort Study			
Author/Year /Country/Ref	Daily Intake	OR/RR	95% CI	Author/Year Country/Ref	Daily Intake	OR/RR	95% CI
Waikens et al. /1996 /USA /[49]	Cases/controls = 271/522 (Men) Q1 Q2 Q3 (Women) Q1 Q2 Q2	1.0 1.1 1.1 1.0 0.8 0.9	0.6–1.9 0.6–2.3 0.3–2.1 0.3–2.6	Chyou et al. /1993 /USA /[50] Nagano et al. /2000 /Japan /[51]	Never Ever 0–1 cup 2–4 ≥ 5	1.0 1.34 1.0 1.07 1.07	0.79–2.27 0.61–2.00 0.58–2.08
Wakai et al. /2004 /Japan /[47]	124/744 < 1–4 5–9 ≥ 10	1.0 1.40 2.67 1.18	0.74–2.62 1.44–4.94 0.49–2.84	Kurahashi et al. /2009 /Japan /[52]	(Men) <1 cup 1–2 3–4 ≥ 5 (Women) <3 3–4 ≥ 5	1.0 1.18 0.71 0.90 1.0 1.22 2.29	0.73–1.91 0.43–1.18 0.56–1.45 0.49–3.00 1.06–4.92
Hemelt et al. /2010 /China /[53]	381/371 0 <Daily Daily <4 ≥ 4	1.00 0.83 1.02 1.23 0.83	0.54–1.27 0.71–1.48 0.76–1.97 0.53–1.28				
Wang et al. /2013 /USA /[49]	1007/1299 Never 0.1–0.13 ≥ 0.14	1.0 0.82 0.60	0.61–1.11 0.45–0.79				

ref: reference. OR: odds ratio. RR: relative ratio. CI: confidential interval.

As shown in Table 1, four of the seven studies were performed in Asian countries. In addition, among the three studies performed in the USA, the subjects were of Japanese ancestry in one and in another were Japanese individuals living in the USA [47,49,50]. Case-control and cohort studies have not been performed in Central and South America, Europe, or Africa. This does not mean that researchers and residents in these countries are not interested in the anticancer effects of tea extracts, including catechins, in bladder cancer. In fact, to clarify the relationship between fluid intake and the risk of urothelial cancer, a multicenter cohort study was designed for 233 and 236 subjects from 23 centers in 10 European countries [54]. The findings of that study revealed that the intake of tea and herbal tea was not associated with the risk of urothelial cancer. However, the effects of green tea per se were not investigated. Moreover, information concerning the anticancer effects of green tea in white and black individuals is scarce.

With regard to epidemiological studies, we should also pay attention to the fact that various units are used to measure green tea consumption, such as frequency/day, cups/day, and mL/day. In addition, the volume per cup differs among countries and regions. For example, the volume of representative cups used for consuming green tea in Japan (120–140 mL) is less than that in Western countries. This information is important when considering the clinical usefulness of green tea. It would be useful if more detailed information about the amount of green tea consumed were included in such reports in future.

3.1.2. Meta-Analyses

There have been several reports of meta-analyses of the relationship between green tea consumption and bladder cancer risk. In this review, we have focused on meta-analyses published in English, because we could not verify the content of publications in other languages. A summary of these meta-analyses is presented in Table 2.

Table 2. Meta-analyses of the relationship between green tea consumption and bladder cancer risk.

Author/Year /Reference	Number of Case-Control Studies	Number of Cohort Studies	Odds Ratio	95% Confidence Interval
Qin et al./2012/[55]	2	3	0.97	0.73–1.21
Wang et al./2013/[13]	2	2	0.81	0.68–0.98
Wu et al./2013/[56]	3	2	1.03	0.82–1.31
Zhang et al./2015/[57]	0	3	1.02	0.95–1.11
Weng et al./2017/[58]	4	3	0.95	0.73–1.24

Only one meta-analysis showed a negative correlation between green tea consumption and bladder cancer risk [13], while the remaining four showed no association between green tea consumption and the risk. A meta-analysis of three cohort studies and three hospital-based case-control studies showed that green tea consumption was not related to a decreased risk of bladder cancer (odds ratio, 0.97; 95% confidential interval, 0.73–1.21) [55]; in addition, another meta-analysis of two cohort studies and three case-control studies showed that there was no significant relationship (relative risk, 1.03; 95% confidential interval, 0.82–1.31) between green tea consumption and bladder cancer risk [56]. Yet, another dose–response meta-analysis of 25 case-control studies and seven prospective cohort studies showed no significant association between green tea consumption and bladder cancer risk [58].

On other hand, it should be noted that the number of studies included in these meta-analyses was relatively small. Although the meta-analysis by Weng et al. assessed the relationship between the consumption of various types of tea (black tea, oolong tea, herbal tea, etc.) and bladder cancer risk in 32 studies (25 case-control studies and seven cohort studies), it included only seven studies involving green tea consumption [58]. Another limitation of these meta-analyses is that they did not include papers published in languages other than English. We found a meta-analysis of five studies showing that increased consumption of green tea may have a protective effect on bladder cancer (odds ratio, 0.76; 95% confidential interval, 0.66–0.95); however, only three of those five studies were verifiable [59]. Considering that green tea is a major beverage for Asians, the majority of whom are not native English speakers, we believe that the publication of English versions of studies published in Asian languages is important.

3.2. Mechanisms Underlying the Anticancer Effects of Green Tea in Bladder Cancer

Although it remains unclear how GTPs regulate malignant aggressiveness, various cancer-related mechanisms and molecules are known to play important roles in the anticancer effects of green tea. In addition, green tea and its extracts have been suggested to affect multiple pathological activities and signaling pathways [60]. Therefore, we evaluated the relationships between GTP and cancer-related functions, including cell survival, cell death, migration, and the cell cycle, in bladder cancer cell lines (Table 3).

Table 3. Relationships between green tea polyphenol treatment and various cancer-related functions in in vitro studies of bladder cancer cell lines.

Cell Line	Type	Dosage/Concentration	Author/Year/Reference
Growth inhibition			
AY-27	EGCG	>100 µM	Kemberling et al./2003/[61]
NBT-II	EGCG	10, 20, or 40 µM/L	Chen et al./2004/[62]
J82	EGCG	70–87 µM	Rieger et al./2007/[63]
UM-UC-3	EGCG	70–87 µM	Rieger et al./2007/[63]
EJ	EGCG	70–87 µM	Rieger et al./2007/[63]
		70–87 µM	Rieger et al./2007/[63];
T24	EGCG	20–100 µg/mL	Qin et al./2007/[64];
		20–80 µg/mL	Philips et al./2009/[65]
KK47	EGCG	70–87 µM	Rieger et al./2007/[63]
TCCSUP	EGCG	70–87 µM	Rieger et al./2007/[63];
		10–80 µg/mL	Philips et al./2009/[65]
TSGH-8301	EGCG	25–100 µM	Chen et al./2011/[66]
MBT-2	EGCG	12.5–50 µM	Hsieh et al./2011/[67]
RT4	EGCG	60–80 µg/mL	Philips et al./2009/[65]
SW780	EGCG	10–80 µg/mL	Philips et al./2009/[65]
Apoptosis induction			
NBT-II	EGCG	10 µM/L	Chen et al./2004/[62]
T24	EGCG	10–80 µg/mL	Qin et al./2007/[64]
TCCSUP	EGCG	40 µg/mL	Philips et al./2009/[65]
TSGH-8301	EGCG	75 µM	Chen et al./2011/[66]
MBT-2	EGCG	50 µM	Hsieh et al./2011/[67]
SW780	EGCG	50–200 µM	Luo et al./2017/[27]
Migration inhibition			
UM-UC-3	EGCG	5 µM	Rieger et al./2007/[63]
EJ	EGCG	5 µM	Rieger et al./2007/[63]
TCCSUP	EGCG	5 µM	Rieger et al./2007/[63]
SW780	EGCG	25–50 µM	Luo et al./2017/[27]
Cell cycle arrest			
NBT-II	EGCG	10, 20, or 40 µM/L	Chen et al./2004/[62]

EGCG: epigallocatechin-3-gallate. GTP: green tea polyphenol.

3.2.1. Cancer Cell Proliferation and Cell Death

In vitro studies have shown that EGCG suppressed cancer cell proliferation and growth in various types of bladder cancer cell lines. Interestingly, one study showed that a high concentration (60 µg/mL) of ECG and ECGC significantly suppressed the proliferation of bladder cancer cell lines (RT4, SW780, TCCSUP, and T24) [65]. However, the same study also showed that a low concentration (10 µg/mL) of ECG could suppress proliferation in SW780, but not in RT4 and T24 [65]. Thus, we speculate that the inhibitory effects of green tea polyphenols on bladder cancer cell proliferation are regulated by complex mechanisms.

In addition to its effects on cancer cell proliferation, EGCG induced apoptosis in various types of bladder cancer cell lines, regardless of the malignant potential and species (Table 3). A study showed that EGCG played an important role in not only the induction of apoptosis, but also the inhibition of growth in a bladder cancer cell line (NBT-II) [62]. However, another study showed that EGCG affected only the apoptosis of bladder cancer cells (SW780), but not cell proliferation or migration [27].

Autophagy is a highly conservative catabolic process used by eukaryotic cells for the degradation of damaged or superfluous proteins and organelles [66]. Although autophagy plays important roles in cell signaling and cellular homeostasis, including physiological cytoprotective or prosurvival mechanisms, completely uncontrolled or excessive autophagy has been associated with cell death [68]. Autophagy is also recognized as an important factor for understanding the pathological characteristics and for planning treatment strategies for many types of cancers [69,70]. This process is stimulated by various stimuli, including nutrients [71,72]. In fact, in bladder cancer cells, autophagy plays an important role in pathological processes and signaling pathways via external stimuli, including natural products [73,74]. With regard to the relationship between autophagy and GTPs, an in vitro study showed that the latter inhibited epirubicin-induced autophagy [75].

Thus, GTPs, especially EGCG, play important roles in cell survival, and affect cell proliferation and cell death in various types of bladder cancer cell lines. On the other hand, as shown in Table 3, the dosage and concentration of EGCG used in in vitro studies varied greatly. Further studies are necessary to judge the optimal dosage and concentration to ascertain the relationship between GTP and bladder cancer cell survival.

3.2.2. Other Cancer-Related Mechanisms

Cancer cell migration and invasion are two key processes for cancer cell dissemination and metastasis in almost all solid tumors, including bladder cancer. As shown in Table 3, in vitro studies have used scratch assays and migration assays to show that EGCG suppressed cell migration and invasion. However, information pertaining to cell migration and invasion is scarce relative to that related to cell survival and death. On the other hand, the concentrations of EGCG that inhibited bladder cancer cell migration were typically lower than those that affected tumor growth and apoptosis (Table 3). More detailed investigations are needed to clarify this issue.

A previous study showed that EGCG caused cell cycle arrest in rat transitional cell cancer [62]. Another study suggested that tea polyphenols can deregulate the cell cycle in bladder cancer cells [46]. Oxidative stress is defined as an imbalance between the cellular production of reactive oxygen species (ROS) and antioxidants; excessive production of ROS causes DNA damage and promotes the activities of oncogenes and/or inhibits tumor suppressor genes [76]. Oxidative stress plays important roles in the aggressiveness of bladder cancer [77]. A previous study has shown that GTPs can protect against oxidative stress in the event of bladder cell death, although this effect was not detected in one of the bladder cancer cell lines (T24) [78].

On the other hand, as shown in Table 3, EGCG has been most widely used for in vitro studies aiming to clarify the relationship between GTPs and various cancer-related functions. Furthermore, other reports have shown that EGCG is the most important component in terms of the health benefits and anticancer effects of green tea [79,80]. Therefore, ECGC has been the focus of discussion in terms of both potential preventative and of therapeutic approaches for bladder cancer.

3.2.3. Cancer-Related Potential Molecular Targets of Green Tea Polyphenols

Next, we evaluate reports on the relationships between GTPs and cancer-related signaling molecules in bladder cancer cell lines (Table 4).

Table 4. Potential molecular targets of green tea polyphenols in bladder cancer cell lines.

Molecules	Cell Line	Author/Year/Reference
Bcl-2 family	T24	Qin et al./2007/61; Gu et al./2017/[68]
	TSGH-8301	Chen et al./2011/[66]
	MBT-2	Hsieh et al./2011/[67]
	SW780	Luo et al./2017/[27]
	BIU87	Gu et al./2017/[68]
Caspase family	TSGH-8301	Chen et al./2011/[66]
	MBT-2	Hsieh et al./2011/[67]
	SW780	Luo et al./2017/[27]
Cyclin D1	NBT-II	Chen et al./2004/[62]
Cyclin-dependent kinase 4/6	NBT-II	Chen et al./2004/[62]
Heat shock protein 27	TSGH-8301	Chen et al./2011/[65]
JNK/Bcl-2/Beclin-1	T24, BIU87	Gu et al./2017/[75]
Matrix metalloproteinase-9	SW780	Luo et al./2017/[27]
N-cadherin	UM-UC-3	Rieger et al./2007/[63]
Nuclear factor-kappa B	TCCSUP	Philips et al./2009/[65]
	SW780	Luo et al./2017/[27]
Phosphatidylinositol 3-kinase /Akt signaling	UM-UC-3	Rieger et al./2007/[63]
	T24	Qin et al./2007/[64]
	TSGH-8301	Chen et al./2011/[66]
Retinoblastoma protein	NBT-II	Chen et al./2004/[62]
Wnt signaling	TCCSUP	Philips et al./2009/[65]

As shown in Table 4, GTPs can regulate the expression and activity of various types of cancer-related molecules. Among them, the bcl-2 and caspase families are well-known important regulators of apoptosis in many types of cancer cells, including bladder cancer cells [81–83]. In addition, phosphatidylinositol 3-kinase (PI3K)/Akt signaling is one of the most important mediators for the regulation of pathological activities such as cell proliferation, apoptosis, and progression in malignancies, including bladder cancer [82,84,85]. Furthermore, a JNK/Bcl-2/Beclin-1-mediated mechanism is associated with autophagy and apoptosis in bladder cancer cells [68]. As a mechanism underlying the pro-apoptotic function, the regulation of nuclear factor-kappa B and matrix metalloproteinase (MMP)-9 has been suggested [27]. Various apoptosis-related molecules have been associated with GTP-induced cell death in bladder cancer cells. Surprisingly, however, there has been no study of the relationship between GTPs and p53 status and function in bladder cancer, even though significant mechanistic associations have been reported in other types of malignancies [86,87]. Therefore, the effects of GTPs on bladder cancer cell proliferation and death require further investigation.

MMP-9 and N-cadherin, which play crucial roles in cancer cell migration and invasion in bladder cancer [88,89], are reportedly modulated by GTPs in bladder cancer cell lines [27,63]. However, there is little information on the effect of GTPs on E-cadherin, which is the best known and classical member of the cadherin family, in bladder cancer. Similarly, the influence of GTPs on MMP-2, which is a strong stimulator of cell invasion and migration, remains unclear. However, there has been a report that a mixture of lysin, proline, arginine, ascorbic acid, and GTEs inhibited cancer cell invasion via the regulation of MMP-2 and MMP-9 production in a bladder cancer cell line (T24) [90].

In a bladder cancer cell line established from Wistar rats (NBT-II), EGCG caused growth inhibition and cell cycle arrest via the downregulation of cyclin D1, cyclin-dependent kinase 4/6, and retinoblastoma protein in terms of regulation of cell cycle progression [62]. As mentioned above, several investigators have reported that GTPs play an important role in cell cycle regulation in bladder cancer cells [46,62]. However, more detailed information on the molecular mechanisms is necessary to understand the antibladder cancer effects of green tea.

Proteomic analysis has shown that EGCG affects the expression levels of heat shock protein 27 in the TSGH-8301 cell line [66]. Interestingly, a recent study showed that heat shock protein 27 expression was significantly associated with clinicopathological features, including the stage and grade, of bladder cancer in 132 patients [91]. The same study also showed no association with clinical outcomes, such as tumor recurrence, progression, and patient survival. Detailed mechanistic links between GTPs and heat shock protein 27 in other diseases, including cancers, have been reported, and knowledge of changes in heat shock protein 27 activities by green tea are important for the evaluation of cancer-related signal pathways and development of new therapeutic strategies [92]. With regard to bladder cancer, more detailed investigations of GTP-induced anticancer effects of heat shock protein 27 are therefore necessary.

In summary, various types of cancer-related molecules are modulated by GTPs. These molecules usually play multiple roles in the malignant behavior of most cancers, including bladder cancer. For example, MMP-9 plays an important role in apoptosis and cell migration, while Wnt signaling plays an important role in cell proliferation, cell cycle regulation, apoptosis, and migration in bladder cancer [93,94]. We propose that identification of detailed molecular mechanisms of anticancer cell effects by GTPs is essential for targeting the key signaling molecules.

3.2.4. Correlation with Genetic Polymorphisms

A previous report has showed that, although the frequency of green tea consumption was not significantly associated with breast cancer risk in all women or in women with the low-activity genotype of the angiotensin-converting enzyme (ACE), a significant decrease in cancer risk with an increase in the frequency of green tea consumption was found in women bearing the high-activity genotype of ACE [95]. Furthermore, the same study group showed that methylenetetrahydrofolate reductase and thymidylate synthase genotypes affected the association between green tea consumption and breast cancer risk [24]. In recent years, several studies on various malignancies have shown the relationship between the anticancer effects of GTPs and genetic polymorphisms [96,97]. With regard to bladder cancer, a study reported that genotype was significantly associated with tea consumption-associated changes in bladder cancer risk [47]. Tea consumption did not decrease the risk of bladder cancer for rs7571337 AA-genotype carriers, whereas it decreased the risk for carriers of the rs7571337 AG+GG genotypes [47]. Unfortunately, the study evaluated the effects of a mix of green tea, black tea, decaffeinated tea, and other herbal teas, rather than those of green tea alone [47]. In another study, lymph node metastasis from urothelial cancer was associated with the methylation status of *DACT1*, which is controlled by polymorphisms in the gene encoding methylenetetrahydrofolate reductase (MTHFR) [98]. Similarly, *MTHFR* 677T polymorphisms were reported to be associated with hypomethylation of insulin-like growth factor-2, the proportion of which was significantly associated with lymph node metastasis [99]. However, such DNA methylation was not significantly associated with green tea consumption [98,99].

In summary, the anticancer effects of GTPs according to genetic polymorphisms in patients with bladder cancer require further studies, with an emphasis on the prevention of carcinogenesis and tumor progression in multiple population groups. Of note, most previous studies were conducted in Asian subjects.

3.3. Anticancer Effects of Green Tea in Animal Models

Various in vivo studies using animal models have shown that GTEs may be useful therapeutic agents for patients with bladder cancer (Table 5).

Table 5. Anticancer effects of green tea in animal models of bladder cancer.

Author/Year/Reference	Agents	Methods	Animal Model	Summary of Results
Sato et al./1999/[100]	GTE	Drinking	Rat; Chemically induced	Dose-dependently inhibited tumor growth when administered after the carcinogen
Sato et al./2003/[101]	GTE	Drinking	Rat; Chemically induced	Prevented tumor growth when administered before the carcinogen
Kemberling et al./2003/[61]	EGCG	Intra-vesical	Rat; intravesical implantation	Inhibited the growth of transitional carcinoma cells
Rieger et al./2007/[63]	EGCG	Drinking	Xenograft model	Over 50% decrease in the mean final tumor volume
Sagara et al./2010/[102]	GTE	Drinking	Mouse; Chemically induced	Inhibited tumor growth and invasion via regulation of angiogenesis
Chen et al./2011/[66]	ECGC	Gavage	Mouse; xenograft model	Inhibited tumor growth in a dose-dependent manner
Hsieh et al./2011/[67]	EGCG	Orally, intraperitoneally, intratumor	Mouse; injection of cancer cells	EGCG–gold nanoparticles were more effective than free EGCG in inhibiting tumor growth
Henriques et al./2014/[103]	Whole green tea	Drinking	Mouse; Chemically induced	Influenced inflammation in the urothelium, but not carcinogenesis
Matsuo et al./2017/[104]	GTE	Drinking	Mouse; Chemically induced	Inhibited tumor growth and angiogenesis via human-antigen R-related pathways

ref: reference. GTEs: green tea extracts. ECGC: epigallocatechin-3-gallate.

While one study reported that GTPs inhibited tumor growth and invasion via regulation of angiogenesis in a mouse model of chemically (N-butyl-N-(4-hydroxybutyl)-nitrosamine; BBN) induced bladder cancer [102], another reported that green tea infusion did not affect the development of bladder cancer after chemical induction in a mouse model [103]. However, the latter study used whole green tea, not GTEs. In another study, GTP intake suppressed the expression of cyclooxygenase-2, hemeoxygenase-1, and human antigen-R (HuR), and this suppression of cancer-related molecules led to the inhibition of cancer cell proliferation and angiogenesis in a mouse model of BBN-induced bladder cancer [104]. Interestingly, the study also found that VEGF-A expression was not directly affected by green tea intake, although it was regulated by green tea intake via HuR regulation [104]. Therefore, green tea intake is speculated to regulate various malignant behaviors through complex mechanisms.

Some rat models of bladder cancer also showed the anticancer effects of green tea. In a study of Fisher 344 rats implanted with urothelial cancer cells (AY-27), 18 of 28 (64%) rats who received intravesical EGCG instillation were free of tumors, whereas all 12 control rats developed tumors [61]. These findings indicated that intravesical EGCG instillation significantly ($p = 0.001$) suppressed the growth of urothelial cell carcinoma in rats [61]. Another study involving a rat model of bladder cancer induced by the intake of drinking water containing BBN showed that the number and volume of tumors were significantly fewer in rats treated with powdered green tea than in control rats that received no such treatment [101]. The same authors also showed dose-dependent anticancer effects of green tea powder intake in a similar rat model of bladder cancer [100]. On the other hand, it has been reported that green tea infusion influences urothelial inflammation, but not carcinogenesis, in a mouse model of BBN-induced bladder cancer [103]. However, in that study, mice treated with BBN only showed no cancer cells.

Taken together, the anticancer effects of GTPs were confirmed in various animal models, and these results support the need for preclinical studies and clinical trials of the use of GTPs in the prevention of recurrence and progression in patients with bladder cancer.

3.4. Bladder Cancer Treatment and Prevention Strategies Based on Green Tea Consumption

Epirubicin is an effective anticancer agent for bladder cancer. Epirubicin reportedly induces this cytoprotective autophagy in bladder cancer cell lines [67]. Interestingly, GTPs inhibited epirubicin-induced autophagy and promoted apoptosis in the same study [67]. Accordingly, it was suggested that GTPs can be used in combination with epirubicin for enhanced epirubicin-based bladder cancer therapy.

Discrepancies in findings regarding the anticancer effects of green tea between epidemiological studies and in vitro studies can be attributed to differences in the concentration of the GTPs used among studies. The concentration of GTPs used in in vivo studies is routinely lower than that used in in vitro studies [105]. In one study, patients with prostate cancer received polyphenon E, which is derived from a hot water extract of green tea leaves (*Camellia sinensis*) and contains 85–95% catechins, including EGCG, for 3–6 weeks before surgery. However, GTP levels in the prostatectomy tissue were low to undetectable [106]. In addition, in a phase II randomized double-blind trial of bladder cancer, polyphenon E or placebo was administered prior to transurethral resection or radical cystectomy, following which tissue EGCG levels were compared between the experimental and placebo groups; there was no significant difference between the two groups [107]. On the basis of these findings, several investigators have shown interest in new technologies and methods that can achieve higher concentrations of GTPs in cancer tissues.

Nanoparticles are recognized as useful drug carriers. The use of EGCG–gold nanoparticles was found to be more effective than the use of free EGCG for treatment in an animal model of bladder cancer [67]. Moreover, EGCG–gold nanoparticles administered orally, intraperitoneally, and intratumorally suppressed tumor growth in C3H/He mice injected with murine bladder cancer cells (MBT-2). The anticancer effects were greater with intraperitoneal and intratumoral administration than with oral administration [67]. Another study showed that Mg(II)-catechin nanocomposite particles had anticancer effects in vitro and in vivo in a rat model of in situ bladder cancer [108]. In that study, Mg(II)-catechin nanocomposite particles that delivered siRNA targeting oncogene eukaryotic translation initiation factor 5A2, showed enhanced antitumor activity [108].

Various new treatment and prevention strategies based on GTPs have been developed in in vitro studies and animal experiments. Some of them have been confirmed to be effective in vivo in bladder cancer animal models. Therefore, there is now a need for translational studies of such in vitro and animal experiments in humans.

3.5. Safety

In general, GTPs are considered to be safe because they are natural compounds. GTPs were found to have no toxic effects on normal cells in the gallbladder [28]. Furthermore, 24-h treatment with 20 µg/mL and 40 µg/mL of EGCG increased the frequency of apoptotic cells in colon cancer cell lines (COLO205), while no significant changes were observed in normal colon epithelial cells (NCM460) [19]. Although green tea and its extracts have a relatively high level of safety for normal cells, it should be noted that "natural" does not always imply safety. In fact, a review on the toxicological effects of green tea showed that various side effects occurred in animal models, healthy volunteers, and patients, with hepatotoxicity, gastrointestinal disorders, and nervous system stimulation being the most important effects, although green tea and its main components are not recognized as major teratogenic, mutagenic, or carcinogenic substances [2]. The study also recommended that green tea should be used with caution in pregnancy, while breast feeding, and in susceptible individuals, as data in these contexts are limited [2].

In normal urothelial cells (UROtsa cell line), GTEs, including ECG and EGCG, were found to inhibit growth in a dose-dependent manner [62]. Another report mentioned that bladder cancer cells (SW780 cell line) were much more sensitive to EGCG than normal bladder epithelial cells (SV-HUC-1 cell line) [27]. In that study, 24-h treatment with EGCG at 100 mM induced cell proliferation inhibition of more than 70% in SW780 cells and of only 7.8% in SV-HUC-1 cells [27]. In addition to anticancer effects, preventive effects against oxidative stress in normal bladder cancer cells have been reported [78].

We previously discussed the anticancer effects of GTPs in a mouse model of BBN-induced bladder cancer [102,104]. When normal urothelial cells in mice treated with GTPs were examined by hematoxylin–eosin staining, abnormal morphological changes were not detected. However, more detailed analyses are necessary to confirm the safety and biological effects of GTPs on normal urothelial cells.

4. Future Direction

The anticancer effects of green tea in bladder cancer have been analyzed using comprehensive methods in epidemiological studies, in vitro studies using bladder cancer cell lines, animal models, and in vivo studies using human tissues. However, some limitations need to be overcome in order to understand the effects of green tea more accurately. Prospective randomized clinical trials with large study populations are yet to be performed to determine the anticancer effects of green tea in Western countries, including the USA, since epidemiological studies have provided some evidence that can serve as a foundation for such trials. On the other hand, such trials are difficult to design because the frequency and amount of green tea consumption in these countries are quite low.

As mentioned above, a combination of conventional chemotherapy and GTPs can be effective in several cancers, including bladder cancer [35,36,67]. In recent years, green tea has come to be known as a radiation sensitizer in prostate cancer [109]. However, there is little information on green tea-induced changes in terms of the anticancer effects of radiotherapy for bladder cancer. At present, immune checkpoint inhibitors are the major therapeutic agents used for patients with advanced/metastatic bladder cancer [110,111], and the usefulness of green tea as a sensitizer of immune checkpoint inhibitors has not yet been investigated. Therefore, more information on the efficacy and safety of combination therapy involving cytotoxic anticancer methods and green tea consumption or GTP intake in bladder cancer is warranted.

Clarification of the extent of the anticancer effects of green tea is difficult, because other bladder cancer-related external factors, such as smoking, exposure to chemical agents, and family history, also play a role [112–115]. In addition, the influence of other beverages, such as coffee, black tea, and oolong tea, and the total fluid intake should be investigated. Furthermore, GTP has complex molecular interactions that could contribute to its potential health benefits [80]. We hope that this review will encourage further investigations of the anticancer effects of green tea that could lead to the development of new treatment and prevention strategies based on green tea consumption and GTP intake, which are relatively safe.

5. Conclusions

In this review, we summarized studies on the potential anticancer effects of green tea consumption and GTP intake in bladder cancer by gathering data from epidemiological, in vivo, and in vitro studies, which have shown conflicting results. In vitro studies using cancer cell lines indicated that GTPs suppress malignant behavior via inhibition of cancer cell proliferation, migration, and invasion and inhibition of apoptosis, and some in vivo studies using animal model also showed similar results. However, some epidemiological studies showed no significant relationship between green tea consumption and the risk of bladder cancer. These discrepancies can be attributed to differences in the race, country, and measurement unit for green tea consumption and/or the influence of other factors, such as smoking, amount of green tea consumption per day, and the intake of other beverages. Therefore, more detailed and wider analyses of larger study populations from various countries, including USA, Europe, and Africa, are necessary to confirm the anticancer effects and usefulness of green tea as an anticancer agent. The anticancer effects of GTPs alone are considered to be limited, whereas a combination of GTPs and other strategies, such as chemotherapy, radiotherapy, immune therapy, and molecular targeted therapy is expected to have some clinical benefit in patients with cancer, including bladder cancer.

Funding: This Review received no external funding.

Acknowledgments: This study was supported in part by a Grant-in-Aid from the Japan Society for the Promotion of Science (to Yasuyoshi Miyata). No private funding was received for this study.

Conflicts of Interest: The authors declare no conflicts of interest.

References

1. Cooper, R.; Morré, D.J.; Morré, D.M. Medicinal benefits of green tea: Part I. Review of noncancer health benefits. *J. Altern. Complement. Med.* **2005**, *11*, 521–528. [CrossRef] [PubMed]
2. Bedrood, Z.; Rameshrad, M.; Hosseinzadeh, H. Toxicological effects of *Camellia sinensis* (green tea): A review. *Phytother. Res.* **2018**, *32*, 1163–1180. [CrossRef] [PubMed]
3. Surh, Y.J. Cancer chemoprevention with dietary phytochemicals. *Nat. Rev. Cancer* **2003**, *3*, 768–780. [CrossRef] [PubMed]
4. Yang, C.S.; Wang, X.; Lu, G.; Picinich, S.C. Cancer prevention by tea: Animal studies, molecular mechanisms and human relevance. *Nat. Rev. Cancer* **2009**, *9*, 429–439. [CrossRef] [PubMed]
5. Bag, A.; Bag, N. Tea polyphenols and prevention of epigenetic aberrations in cancer. *J. Nat. Sci. Biol. Med.* **2018**, *9*, 2–5. [CrossRef] [PubMed]
6. Yang, C.S.; Wang, H.; Li, G.X.; Yang, Z.; Guan, F.; Jin, H. Cancer prevention by tea: Evidence from laboratory studies. *Pharmacol. Res.* **2011**, *64*, 113–122. [CrossRef] [PubMed]
7. Iwasaki, M.; Mizusawa, J.; Kasuga, Y.; Yokoyama, S.; Onuma, H.; Nishimura, H.; Kusama, R.; Tsugane, S. Green tea consumption and breast cancer risk in Japanese women: A case-control study. *Nutr. Cancer* **2014**, *66*, 57–67. [CrossRef] [PubMed]
8. Ogawa, T.; Sawada, N.; Iwasaki, M.; Budhathoki, S.; Hidaka, A.; Yamaji, T.; Shimazu, T.; Sasazuki, S.; Narita, Y.; Tsugane, S. Coffee and green tea consumption in relation to brain tumor risk in a Japanese population. *Int. J. Cancer* **2016**, *139*, 2714–2721. [CrossRef] [PubMed]
9. Zeng, J.L.; Li, Z.H.; Wang, Z.C.; Zhang, H.L. Green tea consumption and risk of pancreatic cancer: A meta-analysis. *Nutrients* **2014**, *6*, 4640–4650. [CrossRef] [PubMed]
10. Sun, C.L.; Yuan, J.M.; Koh, W.P.; Lee, H.P.; Yu, M.C. Green tea and black tea consumption in relation to colorectal cancer risk: The Singapore Chinese Health Study. *Carcinogenesis* **2007**, *28*, 2143–2148. [CrossRef] [PubMed]
11. Oze, I.; Matsuo, K.; Kawakita, D.; Hosono, S.; Ito, H.; Watanabe, M.; Hatooka, S.; Hasegawa, Y.; Shinoda, M.; Tajima, K.; et al. Coffee and green tea consumption is associated with upper aerodigestive tract cancer in Japan. *Int. J. Cancer* **2014**, *135*, 391–400. [CrossRef] [PubMed]
12. Boehm, K.; Borrelli, F.; Ernst, E.; Habacher, G.; Hung, S.K.; Milazzo, S.; Horneber, M. Green tea (*Camellia sinensis*) for the prevention of cancer. *Cochrane Database Syst. Rev.* **2009**, *8*. [CrossRef] [PubMed]
13. Wang, X.; Lin, Y.W.; Wang, S.; Wu, J.; Mao, Q.Q.; Zheng, X.Y.; Xie, L.P. A meta-analysis of tea consumption and the risk of bladder cancer. *Urol. Int.* **2013**, *90*, 10–16. [CrossRef] [PubMed]
14. Tsao, A.S.; Liu, D.; Martin, J.; Tang, X.M.; Lee, J.J.; El-Naggar, A.K.; Wistuba, I.; Culotta, K.S.; Mao, L.; Gillenwater, A.; et al. Phase II randomized, placebo-controlled trial of green tea extract in patients with high-risk oral premalignant lesions. *Cancer Prev. Res.* **2009**, *2*, 931–941. [CrossRef] [PubMed]
15. Singh, B.N.; Shankar, S.; Srivastava, R.K. Green tea catechin, epigallocatechin-3-gallate (EGCG): Mechanisms, perspectives and clinical applications. *Biochem. Pharmacol.* **2011**, *82*, 1807–1821. [CrossRef] [PubMed]
16. Toden, S.; Tran, H.M.; Tovar-Camargo, O.A.; Okugawa, Y.; Goel, A. Epigallocatechin-3-gallate targets cancer stem-like cells and enhances 5-fluorouracil chemosensitivity in colorectal cancer. *Oncotarget* **2016**, *7*, 16158–16171. [CrossRef] [PubMed]
17. Fujiki, H.; Watanabe, T.; Sueoka, E.; Rawangkan, A.; Suganuma, M. Cancer Prevention with Green Tea and Its Principal Constituent, EGCG: From early investigations to current focus on human cancer stem cells. *Mol. Cells* **2018**, *41*, 73–82. [PubMed]
18. Shi, J.; Liu, F.; Zhang, W.; Liu, X.; Lin, B.; Tang, X. Epigallocatechin-3-gallate inhibits nicotine-induced migration and invasion by the suppression of angiogenesis and epithelial-mesenchymal transition in non-small cell lung cancer cells. *Oncol. Rep.* **2015**, *33*, 2972–2980. [CrossRef] [PubMed]
19. Ni, J.; Guo, X.; Wang, H.; Zhou, T.; Wang, X. Differences in the Effects of EGCG on Chromosomal Stability and Cell Growth between Normal and Colon Cancer Cells. *Molecules* **2018**, *23*, 788. [CrossRef] [PubMed]
20. Imai, K.; Suga, K.; Nakachi, K. Cancer-preventive effects of drinking green tea among a Japanese population. *Prev. Med.* **1997**, *26*, 769–775. [CrossRef] [PubMed]

21. Nakachi, K.; Matsuyama, S.; Miyake, S.; Suganuma, M.; Imai, K. Preventive effects of drinking green tea on cancer and cardiovascular disease: epidemiological evidence for multiple targeting prevention. *Biofactors* **2000**, *13*, 49–54. [CrossRef] [PubMed]
22. Bettuzzi, S.; Brausi, M.; Rizzi, F.; Castagnetti, G.; Peracchia, G.; Corti, A. Chemoprevention of human prostate cancer by oral administration of green tea catechins in volunteers with high-grade prostate intraepithelial neoplasia: A preliminary report from a one-year proof-of-principle study. *Cancer Res.* **2006**, *66*, 1234–1240. [CrossRef] [PubMed]
23. Nakachi, K.; Suemasu, K.; Suga, K.; Takeo, T.; Imai, K.; Higashi, Y. Influence of drinking green tea on breast cancer malignancy among Japanese patients. *Jpn. J. Cancer Res.* **1998**, *89*, 254–261. [CrossRef] [PubMed]
24. Inoue, M.; Tajima, K.; Mizutani, M.; Iwata, H.; Iwase, T.; Miura, S.; Hirose, K.; Hamajima, N.; Tominaga, S. Regular consumption of green tea and the risk of breast cancer recurrence: Follow-up study from the Hospital-based Epidemiologic Research Program at Aichi Cancer Center (HERPACC), Japan. *Cancer Lett.* **2001**, *167*, 175–182. [CrossRef]
25. Shimizu, M.; Fukutomi, Y.; Ninomiya, M.; Nagura, K.; Kato, T.; Araki, H.; Suganuma, M.; Fujiki, H.; Moriwaki, H. Green tea extracts for the prevention of metachronous colorectal adenomas: A pilot study. *Cancer Epidemiol. Biomarkers Prev.* **2008**, *17*, 3020–3025. [CrossRef] [PubMed]
26. Taniguchi, S.; Fujiki, H.; Kobayashi, H.; Go, H.; Miyado, K.; Sadano, H.; Shimokawa, R. Effect of (−)-epigallocatechin gallate, the main constituent of green tea, on lung metastasis with mouse B16 melanoma cell lines. *Cancer Lett.* **1992**, *65*, 51–54. [CrossRef]
27. Luo, K.W.; Wei, C.; Lung, W.Y.; Wei, X.Y.; Cheng, B.H.; Cai, Z.M.; Huang, W.R. EGCG inhibited bladder cancer SW780 cell proliferation and migration both in vitro and in vivo via down-regulation of NF-κB and MMP-9. *J. Nutr. Biochem.* **2017**, *41*, 56–64. [CrossRef] [PubMed]
28. Wang, J.; Pan, Y.; Hu, J.; Ma, Q.; Xu, Y.; Zhang, Y.; Zhang, F.; Liu, Y. Tea polyphenols induce S phase arrest and apoptosis in gallbladder cancer cells. *Braz. J. Med. Biol. Res.* **2018**, *51*, 6891. [CrossRef] [PubMed]
29. Liu, L.; Hou, L.; Gu, S.; Zuo, X.; Meng, D.; Luo, M.; Zhang, X.; Huang, S.; Zhao, X. Molecular mechanism of epigallocatechin-3-gallate in human esophageal squamous cell carcinoma in vitro and in vivo. *Oncol. Rep.* **2015**, *33*, 297–303. [CrossRef] [PubMed]
30. Zhu, J.; Jiang, Y.; Yang, X.; Wang, S.; Xie, C.; Li, X.; Li, Y.; Chen, Y.; Wang, X.; Meng, Y.; et al. Wnt/β-catenin pathway mediates (−)-Epigallocatechin-3-gallate (EGCG) inhibition of lung cancer stem cells. *Biochem. Biophys. Res. Commun.* **2017**, *482*, 15–21. [CrossRef] [PubMed]
31. Komori, A.; Yatsunami, J.; Okabe, S.; Abe, S.; Hara, K.; Suganuma, M.; Kim, S.J.; Fujiki, H. Anticarcinogenic activity of green tea polyphenols. *Jpn. J. Clin. Oncol.* **1993**, *23*, 186–190. [PubMed]
32. Lecumberri, E.; Dupertuis, Y.M.; Miralbell, R.; Pichard, C. Green tea polyphenol epigallocatechin-3-gallate (EGCG) as adjuvant in cancer therapy. *Clin. Nutr.* **2013**, *32*, 894–903. [CrossRef] [PubMed]
33. Chen, L.; Ye, H.L.; Zhang, G.; Yao, W.M.; Chen, X.Z.; Zhang, F.C.; Liang, G. Autophagy inhibition contributes to the synergistic interaction between EGCG and doxorubicin to kill the hepatoma Hep3B cells. *PLoS ONE* **2014**, *9*, 85771. [CrossRef] [PubMed]
34. Esmaeili, M.A. Combination of siRNA-directed gene silencing with epigallocatechin-3-gallate (EGCG) reverses drug resistance in human breast cancer cells. *J. Chem. Biol.* **2015**, *9*, 41–52. [CrossRef] [PubMed]
35. Suganuma, M.; Saha, A.; Fujiki, H. New cancer treatment strategy using combination of green tea catechins and anticancer drugs. *Cancer Sci.* **2011**, *102*, 317–323. [CrossRef] [PubMed]
36. Fujiki, H.; Sueoka, E.; Watanabe, T.; Suganuma, M. Primary cancer prevention by green tea, and tertiary cancer prevention by the combination of green tea catechins and anticancer compounds. *J. Cancer Prev.* **2015**, *20*, 1–4. [CrossRef] [PubMed]
37. Wang, W.; Chen, D.; Zhu, K. SOX2OT variant 7 contributes to the synergistic interaction between EGCG and Doxorubicin to kill osteosarcoma via autophagy and stemness inhibition. *J. Exp. Lin. Cancer Res.* **2018**, *37*, 37. [CrossRef] [PubMed]
38. Calgarotto, A.K.; Maso, V.; Junior, G.C.F.; Nowill, A.E.; Filho, P.L.; Vassallo, J.; Saad, S.T.O. Antitumor activities of Quercetin and Green Tea in xenografts of human leukemia HL60 cells. *Sci. Rep.* **2018**, *8*, 3459. [CrossRef] [PubMed]
39. Wang, P.; Henning, S.M.; Heber, D.; Vadgama, J.V. Sensitization to docetaxel in prostate cancer cells by green tea and quercetin. *J. Nutr. Biochem.* **2015**, *26*, 408–415. [CrossRef] [PubMed]

40. Chung, J.E.; Tan, S.; Gao, S.J.; Yongvongsoontorn, N.; Kim, S.H.; Lee, J.H.; Choi, H.S.; Yano, H.; Zhuo, L.; Kurisawa, M.; et al. Self-assembled micellar nanocomplexes comprising green tea catechin derivatives and protein drugs for cancer therapy. *Nat. Nanotechnol.* **2014**, *9*, 907–912. [CrossRef] [PubMed]
41. Liang, K.; Chung, J.E.; Gao, S.J.; Yongvongsoontorn, N.; Kurisawa, M. Highly Augmented Drug Loading and Stability of Micellar Nanocomplexes Composed of Doxorubicin and Poly(ethylene glycol)-Green Tea Catechin Conjugate for Cancer Therapy. *Adv. Mater.* **2018**, *30*, 1706963. [CrossRef] [PubMed]
42. Chavan, S.; Bray, F.; Lortet-Tieulent, J.; Goodman, M.; Jemal, A. International variations in bladder cancer incidence and mortality. *Eur. Urol.* **2014**, *66*, 59–73. [CrossRef] [PubMed]
43. Abufaraj, M.; Gust, K.; Moschini, M.; Foerster, B.; Soria, F.; Mathieu, R.; Shariat, S.F. Management of muscle invasive, locally advanced and metastatic urothelial carcinoma of the bladder: A literature review with emphasis on the role of surgery. *Transl. Androl. Urol.* **2016**, *5*, 735–744. [CrossRef] [PubMed]
44. Xu, C.; Zeng, X.T.; Liu, T.Z.; Zhang, C.; Yang, Z.H.; Li, S.; Chen, X.Y. Fruits and vegetables intake and risk of bladder cancer: A PRISMA-compliant systematic review and dose-response meta-analysis of prospective cohort studies. *Medicine (Baltimore)* **2015**, *94*, 759. [CrossRef] [PubMed]
45. Philippou, Y.; Hadjipavlou, M.; Khan, S.; Rane, A. Complementary and alternative medicine (CAM) in prostate and bladder cancer. *BJU Int.* **2013**, *112*, 1073–1079. [CrossRef] [PubMed]
46. Conde, V.R.; Alves, M.G.; Oliveira, P.F.; Silva, B.M. Tea (*Camellia sinensis* (L.)): A putative anticancer agent in bladder carcinoma? *Anticancer Agents Med. Chem.* **2015**, *15*, 26–36. [CrossRef] [PubMed]
47. Wang, J.; Wu, X.; Kamat, A.; Barton, G.H.; Dinney, C.P.; Lin, J. Fluid intake, genetic variants of UDP-glucuronosyltransferases, and bladder cancer risk. *Br. J. Cancer* **2013**, *108*, 2372–2380. [CrossRef] [PubMed]
48. Wakai, K.; Hirose, K.; Takezaki, T.; Hamajima, N.; Ogura, Y.; Nakamura, S.; Hayashi, N.; Tajima, K. Foods and beverages in relation to urothelial cancer: Case-control study in Japan. *Int. J. Urol.* **2004**, *11*, 11–19. [CrossRef] [PubMed]
49. Wilkens, L.R.; Kadir, M.M.; Kolonel, L.N.; Nomura, A.M.; Hankin, J.H. Risk factors for lower urinary tract cancer: the role of total fluid consumption, nitrites and nitrosamines, and selected foods. *Cancer Epidemiol. Biomarkers Prev.* **1996**, *5*, 161–166. [PubMed]
50. Chyou, P.H.; Nomura, A.M.; Stemmermann, G.N. A prospective study of diet, smoking, and lower urinary tract cancer. *Ann. Epidemiol.* **1993**, *3*, 211–216. [CrossRef]
51. Nagano, J.; Kono, S.; Preston, D.L.; Moriwaki, H.; Sharp, G.B.; Koyama, K.; Mabuchi, K. Bladder-cancer incidence in relation to vegetable and fruit consumption: a prospective study of atomic-bomb survivors. *Int. J. Cancer* **2000**, *86*, 132–138. [CrossRef]
52. Kurahashi, N.; Inoue, M.; Iwasaki, M.; Sasazuki, S.; Tsugane, S. Coffee, green tea, and caffeine consumption and subsequent risk of bladder cancer in relation to smoking status: A prospective study in Japan. *Cancer Sci.* **2009**, *100*, 284–291. [CrossRef] [PubMed]
53. Hemelt, M.; Hu, Z.; Zhong, Z.; Xie, L.P.; Wong, Y.C.; Tam, P.C.; Cheng, K.K.; Ye, Z.; Bi, X.; Lu, Q.; et al. Fluid intake and the risk of bladder cancer: Results from the South and East China case-control study on bladder cancer. *Int. J. Cancer* **2010**, *127*, 638–645. [CrossRef] [PubMed]
54. Ros, M.M.; Bas Bueno-de-Mesquita, H.B.; Büchner, F.L.; Aben, K.K.; Kampman, E.; Egevad, L.; Overvad, K.; Tjønneland, A.; Roswall, N.; Clavel-Chapelon, F. Fluid intake and the risk of urothelial cell carcinomas in the European Prospective Investigation into Cancer and Nutrition (EPIC). *Int. J. Cancer* **2011**, *128*, 2695–2708. [CrossRef] [PubMed]
55. Qin, J.; Xie, B.; Mao, Q.; Kong, D.; Lin, Y.; Zheng, X. Tea consumption and risk of bladder cancer: A meta-analysis. *World J. Surg. Oncol.* **2012**, *10*, 172. [CrossRef] [PubMed]
56. Wu, S.; Li, F.; Huang, X.; Hua, Q.; Huang, T.; Liu, Z.; Liu, Z.; Zhang, Z.; Liao, C.; Chen, Y.; et al. The association of tea consumption with bladder cancer risk: A meta-analysis. *Asia Pac. J. Clin. Nutr.* **2013**, *22*, 128–137. [PubMed]
57. Zhang, Y.F.; Xu, Q.; Lu, J.; Wang, P.; Zhang, H.W.; Zhou, L.; Ma, X.Q.; Zhou, Y.H. Tea consumption and the incidence of cancer: A systematic review and meta-analysis of prospective observational studies. *Eur. J. Cancer Prev.* **2015**, *24*, 353–362. [CrossRef] [PubMed]
58. Weng, H.; Zeng, X.T.; Li, S.; Kwong, J.S.; Liu, T.Z.; Wang, X.H. Tea Consumption and Risk of Bladder Cancer: A Dose-Response Meta-Analysis. *Front. Physiol.* **2017**, *7*, 693. [CrossRef] [PubMed]

59. Bai, Y.; Yuan, H.; Li, J.; Tang, Y.; Pu, C.; Han, P. Relationship between bladder cancer and total fluid intake: A meta-analysis of epidemiological evidence. *World J. Surg. Oncol.* **2014**, *12*, 223. [CrossRef] [PubMed]
60. Khan, N.; Afaq, F.; Saleem, M.; Ahmad, N.; Mukhtar, H. Targeting multiple signaling pathways by green tea polyphenol (−)-epigallocatechin-3-gallate. *Cancer Res.* **2006**, *66*, 2500–2505. [CrossRef] [PubMed]
61. Kemberling, J.K.; Hampton, J.A.; Keck, R.W.; Gomez, M.A.; Selman, S.H. Inhibition of bladder tumor growth by the green tea derivative epigallocatechin-3-gallate. *J. Urol.* **2003**, *170*, 773–776. [CrossRef] [PubMed]
62. Chen, J.J.; Ye, Z.Q.; Koo, M.W. Growth inhibition and cell cycle arrest effects of epigallocatechin gallate in the NBT-II bladder tumour cell line. *BJU Int.* **2004**, *93*, 1082–1086. [CrossRef] [PubMed]
63. Rieger-Christ, K.M.; Hanley, R.; Lodowsky, C.; Bernier, T.; Vemulapalli, P.; Roth, M.; Kim, J.; Yee, A.S.; Le, S.M.; Marie, P.J.; et al. The green tea compound, (−)-epigallocatechin-3-gallate downregulates N-cadherin and suppresses migration of bladder carcinoma cells. *J. Cell Biochem.* **2007**, *102*, 377–388. [CrossRef] [PubMed]
64. Qin, J.; Xie, L.P.; Zheng, X.Y.; Wang, Y.B.; Bai, Y.; Shen, H.F.; Li, L.C.; Dahiya, R. A component of green tea, (-)-epigallocatechin-3-gallate, promotes apoptosis in T24 human bladder cancer cells via modulation of the PI3K/Akt pathway and Bcl-2 family proteins. *Biochem. Biophys. Res. Commun.* **2007**, *354*, 852–857. [CrossRef] [PubMed]
65. Philips, B.J.; Coyle, C.H.; Morrisroe, S.N.; Chancellor, M.B.; Yoshimura, N. Induction of apoptosis in human bladder cancer cells by green tea catechins. *Biomed. Res.* **2009**, *4*, 207–215. [CrossRef]
66. Chen, N.G.; Lu, C.C.; Lin, Y.H.; Shen, W.C.; Lai, C.H.; Ho, Y.J.; Chung, J.G.; Lin, T.H.; Lin, Y.C.; Yang, J.S. Proteomic approaches to study epigallocatechin gallate-provoked apoptosis of TSGH-8301 human urinary bladder carcinoma cells: Roles of AKT and heat shock protein 27-modulated intrinsic apoptotic pathways. *Oncol. Rep.* **2011**, *26*, 939–947. [PubMed]
67. Hsieh, D.S.; Wang, H.; Tan, S.W.; Huang, Y.H.; Tsai, C.Y.; Yeh, M.K.; Wu, C.J. The treatment of bladder cancer in a mouse model by epigallocatechin-3-gallate-gold nanoparticles. *Biomaterials* **2011**, *32*, 7633–7640. [CrossRef] [PubMed]
68. Galluzzi, L.; Morselli, E.; Vicencio, J.M.; Kepp, O.; Joza, N.; Tajeddine, N.; Kroemer, G. Life, death and burial: Multifaceted impact of autophagy. *Biochem. Soc. Trans.* **2008**, *36*, 786–790. [CrossRef] [PubMed]
69. Dower, C.M.; Wills, C.A.; Frisch, S.M.; Wang, H.G. Mechanisms and context underlying the role of autophagy in cancer metastasis. *Autophagy* **2018**, in press. [CrossRef] [PubMed]
70. Wilde, L.; Tanson, K.; Curry, J.; Martinez-Outschoorn, U. Autophagy in cancer: A complex relationship. *Biochem. J.* **2018**, *475*, 1939–1954. [CrossRef] [PubMed]
71. Kroemer, G.; Mariño, G.; Levine, B. Autophagy and the integrated stress response. *Mol. Cell* **2010**, *40*, 280–293. [CrossRef] [PubMed]
72. Liuzzi, J.P.; Guo, L.; Yoo, C.; Stewart, T.S. Zinc and autophagy. *BioMetals* **2014**, *27*, 1087–1096. [CrossRef] [PubMed]
73. Fan, B.; Zhang, X.; Ma, Y.; Zhang, A. Fangchinoline Induces Apoptosis, Autophagy and Energetic Impairment in Bladder Cancer. *Cell Physiol. Biochem.* **2017**, *43*, 1003–1011. [CrossRef] [PubMed]
74. Kou, B.; Liu, W.; Xu, X.; Yang, Y.; Yi, Q.; Guo, F.; Li, J.; Zhou, J.; Kou, Q. Autophagy induction enhances tetrandrine-induced apoptosis via the AMPK/mTOR pathway in human bladder cancer cells. *Oncol. Rep.* **2017**, *38*, 3137–3143. [CrossRef] [PubMed]
75. Gu, W.; Lin, Y.; Gou, X.; He, W. Tea Polyphenol inhibits autophagy to sensitize Epirubicin-induced apoptosis in human bladder cancer cells. *Neoplasma* **2017**, *64*, 674–680. [CrossRef] [PubMed]
76. Sies, H. Oxidative stress: Oxidants and antioxidants. *Exp. Physiol.* **1997**, *82*, 291–295. [CrossRef] [PubMed]
77. Miyata, Y.; Matsuo, T.; Sagara, Y.; Ohba, K.; Ohyama, K.; Sakai, H. A Mini-Review of Reactive Oxygen Species in Urological Cancer: Correlation with NADPH Oxidases, Angiogenesis, and Apoptosis. *Int. J. Mol. Sci.* **2017**, *18*, 2214. [CrossRef] [PubMed]
78. Coyle, C.H.; Philips, B.J.; Morrisroe, S.N.; Chancellor, M.B.; Yoshimura, N. Antioxidant effects of green tea and its polyphenols on bladder cells. *Life Sci.* **2008**, *83*, 12–18. [CrossRef] [PubMed]
79. Haque, I.; Subramanian, A.; Huang, C.H.; Godwin, A.K.; Van Veldhuizen, P.J.; Banerjee, S.; Banerjee, S.K. The Role of Compounds Derived from Natural Supplement as Anticancer Agents in Renal Cell Carcinoma: A Review. *Int. J. Mol. Sci.* **2017**, *19*, 107. [CrossRef] [PubMed]
80. Saeki, K.; Hayakawa, S.; Nakano, S.; Ito, S.; Oishi, Y.; Suzuki, Y.; Isemura, M. In Vitro and In Silico Studies of the Molecular Interactions of Epigallocatechin-3-O-gallate (EGCG) with Proteins That Explain the Health Benefits of Green Tea. *Molecules* **2018**, *23*, 1295. [CrossRef] [PubMed]

81. Duggan, B.J.; Gray, S.; Johnston, S.R.; Williamson, K.; Miyaki, H.; Gleave, M. The role of antisense oligonucleotides in the treatment of bladder cancer. *Urol. Res.* **2002**, *30*, 137–147. [CrossRef] [PubMed]
82. Shin, D.Y.; Kim, G.Y.; Hwang, H.J.; Kim, W.J.; Choi, Y.H. Diallyl trisulfide-induced apoptosis of bladder cancer cells is caspase-dependent and regulated by PI3K/Akt and JNK pathways. *Environ. Toxicol. Pharmacol.* **2014**, *37*, 74–83. [CrossRef] [PubMed]
83. Campbell, K.J.; Tait, S.W.G. Targeting BCL-2 regulated apoptosis in cancer. *Open Biol.* **2018**, *8*, 180002. [CrossRef] [PubMed]
84. Wu, X.; Obata, T.; Khan, Q.; Highshaw, R.A.; De Vere White, R.; Sweeney, C. The phosphatidylinositol-3 kinase pathway regulates bladder cancer cell invasion. *BJU Int.* **2004**, *93*, 143–150. [CrossRef] [PubMed]
85. Ahn, K.I.; Choi, E.O.; Kwon, D.H.; HwangBo, H.; Kim, M.Y.; Kim, H.J.; Ji, S.Y.; Hong, S.H.; Jeong, J.W.; Park, C.; et al. Induction of apoptosis by ethanol extract of Citrus unshiu Markovich peel in human bladder cancer T24 cells through ROS-mediated inactivation of the PI3K/Akt pathway. *Biosci. Trends* **2017**, *11*, 565–573. [CrossRef] [PubMed]
86. Fang, C.Y.; Wu, C.C.; Hsu, H.Y.; Chuang, H.Y.; Huang, S.Y.; Tsai, C.H.; Chang, Y.; Tsao, G.S.; Chen, C.L.; Chen, J.Y. EGCG inhibits proliferation, invasiveness and tumor growth by up-regulation of adhesion molecules, suppression of gelatinases activity, and induction of apoptosis in nasopharyngeal carcinoma cells. *Int. J. Mol. Sci.* **2015**, *16*, 2530–2558. [CrossRef] [PubMed]
87. Prasad, R.; Katiyar, S.K. Polyphenols from green tea inhibit the growth of melanoma cells through inhibition of class I histone deacetylases and induction of DNA damage. *Gene. Cancer.* **2015**, *6*, 49–61.
88. Bryan, R.T. Cell adhesion and urothelial bladder cancer: the role of cadherin switching and related phenomena. *Philos. Trans R. Soc. Lond B Biol. Sci.* **2015**, *370*. [CrossRef] [PubMed]
89. Wu, G.J.; Bao, J.S.; Yue, Z.J.; Zeng, F.C.; Cen, S.; Tang, Z.Y.; Kang, X.L. Elevated expression of matrix metalloproteinase-9 is associated with bladder cancer pathogenesis. *J Cancer Res. Ther.* **2018**, *14*, 54–59.
90. Roomi, M.W.; Ivanov, V.; Kalinovsky, T.; Niedzwiecki, A.; Rath, M. Antitumor effect of ascorbic acid, lysine, proline, arginine, and green tea extract on bladder cancer cell line T-24. *Int. J. Urol.* **2006**, *4*, 415–419. [CrossRef] [PubMed]
91. Lee, M.S.; Lee, J.; Lee, S.; Yoo, S M.; Kim, J.H.; Kim, W.T.; Kim, W.J.; Park, J. Clinical, prognostic, and therapeutic significance of heat shock protein 27 in bladder cancer. *Oncotarget* **2018**, *9*, 7961–7974. [CrossRef] [PubMed]
92. Zhang, L.; Pang, E.; Loo, R.R.; Rao, J.; Go, V.L.; Loo, J.A.; Lu, Q.Y. Concomitant inhibition of HSP90, its mitochondrial localized homologue TRAP1 and HSP27 by green tea in pancreatic cancer HPAF-II cells. *Proteomics* **2011**, *11*, 4638–4647. [CrossRef] [PubMed]
93. Casadevall, D.; Kilian, A.Y.; Bellmunt, J. The prognostic role of epigenetic dysregulation in bladder cancer: A systematic review. *Cancer Treat. Rev.* **2017**, *61*, 82–93. [CrossRef] [PubMed]
94. Yoshida, T.; Sopko, N.A.; Kates, M.; Liu, X.; Joice, G.; McConkey, D.J.; Bivalacqua, T.J. Three-dimensional organoid culture reveals involvement of Wnt/β-catenin pathway in proliferation of bladder cancer cells. *Oncotarget* **2018**, *9*, 11060–11070. [CrossRef] [PubMed]
95. Yuan, J.M.; Koh, W.P.; Sun, C.L.; Lee, H.P.; Yu, M.C. Green tea intake, ACE gene polymorphism and breast cancer risk among Chinese women in Singapore. *Carcinogenesis* **2005**, *26*, 1389–1394. [CrossRef] [PubMed]
96. Liu, P.; Zhang, M.; Xie, X.; Jin, J.; Holman, C.D. Green tea consumption and glutathione S-transferases genetic polymorphisms on the risk of adult leukemia. *Eur. J. Nutr.* **2017**, *56*, 603–612. [CrossRef] [PubMed]
97. Scholl, C.; Lepper, A.; Lehr, T.; Hanke, N.; Schneider, K.L.; Brockmöller, J.; Seufferlein, T.; Stingl, J.C. Population nutrikinetics of green tea extract. *PLoS ONE* **2018**, *13*, 0193074. [CrossRef] [PubMed]
98. Cheng, H.; Lu, M.; Mao, L.J.; Wang, J.Q.; Li, W.; Wen, R.M.; Chen, J.C. Relationships among MTHFR a1298c gene polymorphisms and methylation status of Dact1 gene in transitional cell carcinomas. *Asian Pac. J. Cancer Prev.* **2012**, *13*, 5069–5074. [CrossRef] [PubMed]
99. Cheng, H.; Deng, Z.; Wang, Z.; Zhang, W.; Su, J. MTHFR C677T polymorphisms are associated with aberrant methylation of the IGF-2 gene in transitional cell carcinoma of the bladder. *J. Biomed. Res.* **2012**, *26*, 77–83. [CrossRef]
100. Sato, D. Inhibition of urinary bladder tumors induced by N-butyl-N-(4-hydroxybutyl)-nitrosamine in rats by green tea. *Int. J. Urol.* **1999**, *6*, 93–99. [CrossRef] [PubMed]
101. Sato, D.; Matsushima, M. Preventive effects of urinary bladder tumors induced by N-butyl-N-(4-hydroxybutyl)-nitrosamine in rat by green tea leaves. *Int. J. Urol.* **2003**, *10*, 160–166. [CrossRef] [PubMed]

102. Sagara, Y.; Miyata, Y.; Nomata, K.; Hayashi, T.; Kanetake, H. Green tea polyphenol suppresses tumor invasion and angiogenesis in *N*-butyl-(-4-hydroxybutyl) nitrosamine-induced bladder cancer. *Cancer Epidemiol.* **2010**, *34*, 350–354. [CrossRef] [PubMed]
103. Henriques, A.; Arantes-Rodrigues, R.; Faustino-Rocha, A.I.; Teixeira-Guedes, C.I.; Pinho-Oliveira, J.; Talhada, D.; Teixeira, J.H.; Andrade, A.; Colaço, B.; Paiva-Cardoso, M.N.; et al. The effects of whole green tea infusion on mouse urinary bladder chemical carcinogenesis. *Iran. J. Basic Med. Sci.* **2014**, *17*, 145–148. [PubMed]
104. Matsuo, T.; Miyata, Y.; Asai, A.; Sagara, Y.; Furusato, B.; Fukuoka, J.; Sakai, H. Green Tea Polyphenol Induces Changes in Cancer-Related Factors in an Animal Model of Bladder Cancer. *PLoS ONE* **2017**, *12*, 0171091. [CrossRef] [PubMed]
105. Bailey, H.H.; Mukhtar, H. Green tea polyphenols and cancer chemoprevention of genitourinary cancer. *Am. Soc. Clin. Oncol. Educ. Book* **2013**, 92–96. [CrossRef] [PubMed]
106. Nguyen, M.M.; Ahmann, F.R.; Nagle, R.B.; Hsu, C.H.; Tangrea, J.A.; Parnes, H.L.; Sokoloff, M.H.; Gretzer, M.B.; Chow, H.H. Randomized, double-blind, placebo-controlled trial of polyphenon E in prostate cancer patients before prostatectomy: evaluation of potential chemopreventive activities. *Cancer Prev. Res.* **2012**, *5*, 290–298. [CrossRef] [PubMed]
107. Gee, J.R.; Saltzstein, D.R.; Kim, K.; Kolesar, J.; Huang, W.; Havighurst, T.C.; Wollmer, B.W.; Stublaski, J.; Downs, T.; Mukhtar, H.; et al. A Phase II Randomized, Double-blind, Presurgical Trial of Polyphenon E in Bladder Cancer Patients to Evaluate Pharmacodynamics and Bladder Tissue Biomarkers. *Cancer Prev. Res.* **2017**, *10*, 298–307. [CrossRef] [PubMed]
108. Chen, Z.; Yu, T.; Zhou, B.; Wei, J.; Fang, Y.; Lu, J.; Guo, L.; Chen, W.; Liu, Z.P.; Luo, J. Mg(II)-Catechin nanoparticles delivering siRNA targeting EIF5A2 inhibit bladder cancer cell growth in vitro and in vivo. *Biomaterials* **2016**, *81*, 125–134. [CrossRef] [PubMed]
109. Schroeder, A.C.; Xiao, H.; Zhu, Z.; Li, Q.; Bai, Q.; Wakefield, M.R.; Mann, J.D.; Fang, Y. A Potential Role for Green Tea as a Radiation Sensitizer for Prostate Cancer. *Pathol. Oncol. Res.* **2017**, in press. [CrossRef] [PubMed]
110. Bellmunt, J.; de Wit, R.; Vaughn, D.J.; Fradet, Y.; Lee, J.L.; Fong, L.; Vogelzang, N.J.; Climent, M.A.; Petrylak, D.P.; Choueiri, T.K.; et al. Pembrolizumab as second-line therapy for advanced urothelial carcinoma. *N. Engl. J. Med.* **2017**, *376*, 1015–1026. [CrossRef] [PubMed]
111. Rouanne, M.; Roumiguié, M.; Houédé, N.; Masson-Lecomte, A.; Colin, P.; Pignot, G.; Larré, S.; Xylinas, E.; Rouprêt, M.; Neuzillet, Y. Development of immunotherapy in bladder cancer: present and future on targeting PD(L)1 and CTLA-4 pathways. *World J. Urol.* **2018**, in press. [CrossRef] [PubMed]
112. Meyer, J.; Rohrmann, S.; Bopp, M.; Faeh, D. Swiss National Cohort Study Group. Impact of smoking and excess body weight on overall and site-specific cancer mortality risk. *Cancer Epidemiol. Biomarkers Prev.* **2015**, *24*, 1516–1522. [CrossRef] [PubMed]
113. Aben, K.K.; Witjes, J.A.; Schoenberg, M.P.; Hulsbergen-van de, K.C.; Verbeek, A.L.; Kiemeney, L.A. Familial aggregation of urothelial cell carcinoma. *Int. J. Cancer* **2002**, *98*, 274–278. [CrossRef] [PubMed]
114. Espina, C.; Straif, K.; Friis, S.; Kogevinas, M.; Saracci, R.; Vainio, H.; Schüz, J. European Code against Cancer 4th Edition: Environment, occupation and cancer. *Cancer Epidemiol.* **2015**, *39*, 84–92. [CrossRef] [PubMed]
115. Wu, W.; Tong, Y.; Zhao, Q.; Yu, G.; Wei, X.; Lu, Q. Coffee consumption and bladder cancer: a meta-analysis of observational studies. *Sci. Rep.* **2015**, *5*, 9051. [CrossRef] [PubMed]

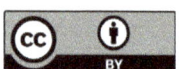

© 2018 by the authors. Licensee MDPI, Basel, Switzerland. This article is an open access article distributed under the terms and conditions of the Creative Commons Attribution (CC BY) license (http://creativecommons.org/licenses/by/4.0/).

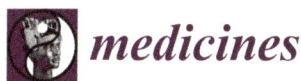

Review

MiR-663, a MicroRNA Linked with Inflammation and Cancer That Is under the Influence of Resveratrol

Jean-Jacques Michaille [1], Victoria Piurowski [2], Brooke Rigot [3], Hesham Kelani [4], Emily C. Fortman [4] and Esmerina Tili [3,4,*]

1. BioPerox-IL, UB-INSERM IFR #100, Faculté Gabriel, Université de Bourgogne-Franche Comté, 21000 Dijon, France; Jean-Jacques.Michaille@u-bourgogne.fr
2. Department of Biology, Franklin College of Arts and Sciences, University of Georgia, Athes, GA 30602, USA; victoria.piurowski@uga.edu
3. Department of Cancer Biology and Genetics, Wexner Medical Center, The Ohio State University, Columbus, OH 43210, USA; rigot.10@buckeyemail.osu.edu
4. Department of Anesthesiology, Wexner Medical Center, The Ohio State University, Columbus, OH 43210, USA; Hesham.Kelani@osumc.edu (H.K.); fortman.64@buckeyemail.osu.edu (E.C.F.)
* Correspondence: Esmerina.Tili@osumc.edu; Tel.: +1-614-688-8042

Received: 8 May 2018; Accepted: 5 July 2018; Published: 9 July 2018

Abstract: Resveratrol (trans-3,5,4′-trihydroxystilbene, RSV) is a non-flavonoid dietary polyphenol with antioxidant, anti-inflammatory and anti-cancer properties that is primarily found in red berries. While RSV displays many beneficial effects in vitro, its actual effects in vivo or in animal models remain passionately debated. Recent publications suggest that RSV pleiotropic effects could arise from its capability to regulate the expression and activity of microRNAs, short regulators themselves capable of regulating up to several hundreds of target genes. In particular, RSV increases microRNA *miR-663* expression in different human cell lines, suggesting that at least some of its multiple beneficial properties are through the modulation of expression of this microRNA. Indeed, the expression of microRNA *miR-663* is reduced in certain cancers where *miR-663* is considered to act as a tumor suppressor gene, as well as in other pathologies such as cardiovascular disorders. Target of *miR-663* include genes involved in tumor initiation and/or progression as well as genes involved in pathologies associated with chronic inflammation. Here, we review the direct and indirect effects of RSV on the expression of *miR-663* and its target transcripts, with emphasise on *TGFβ1*, and their expected health benefits, and argue that elucidating the molecular effects of different classes of natural compounds on the expression of microRNAs should help to identify new therapeutic targets and design new treatments.

Keywords: resveratrol; *miR-663*; inflammation; cancer; cardiovascular disease

1. Introduction

Recent years have brought an increasing number of publications describing the potentials of plant natural products to be used for the treatment of human pathologies. Among those molecules, Resveratrol (trans-3,5,4′-trihydroxystilbene, RSV), which is produced by plants in defense against the pathogen *Botrytis cinerea* [1], is in particular found in the skins of black and red berries. RSV presents strong antioxidant, anti-inflammatory and anti-cancer properties [2,3]. While most of these properties have been demonstrated using cell cultures, RSV precise molecular effects in vivo have remained controversial, in particular because the bioactivity of this compound is limited by the fact that it is rapidly metabolized [4]. Finally, whether resveratrol alone is beneficial to the health, or whether resveratrol metabolites actually participate in delivering beneficial effects, also remains a matter of debate (discussed in [5]).

Pre-clinical studies, however, are presently being conducted to determine the true therapeutic potentials of RSV in the treatment of cancer and cardiovascular diseases [3–8]. On the one hand, several promising results have been reported. For example, the potentials of RSV as a phytoestrogen, an inhibitor of aromatase activity and an adjuvant has been explored in the context of breast cancer [3]. Other studies have been conducted in patients with colorectal, multiple myeloma neuroendocrine tumors, with variable results [7,8]. Beneficial effects of RSV on patients with neurologic, metabolic, and cardiovascular pathologies have also been reported [6,9–12]. Thus, in animal models, resveratrol has been shown to be anti-hypertensive, to modulate the levels of HDLs and LDLs in rats subjected to high fat diet, to reduce myocardial ischemia and ischemia-reperfusion injury, and to reduce cardiac hypertrophy; however, several studies have reported no RSV effect in each type of pathologies (reviewed by [5]).

The biggest challenge finally rests on determining the molecular pathways through which RSV acts in different pathological contexts, determining the optimal RSV dose, the best mode of RSV delivery, and how to increase the bioavailability of RSV in different tissues (discussed in [6]). Based on studies conducted in animal models such as swine, mouse or monkeys, the absorption of regular, low doses of RSV seems to bear promising potentials for preventive therapeutics [6]. Transferring these results in human, however, remains particularly challenging, in particular when it comes to measuring RSV protecting effects in healthy subjects, given in particular the impossibility of conducting long or very long-term studies, that, beyond considerable cost, carry high risks of bias [6]. Thus, while beneficial effects have been reported following RSV treatment of patients that were either healthy, obese or presenting different pathologies associated with the metabolic syndrome, other studies reported a lack of effects of this molecule (discussed by [6]).

One fact could potentially explain the apparent paradox of a molecule with low biological availability providing pleiotropic beneficial effects in many different contexts: it is that RSV can globally change the composition of endogenous microRNA populations [13]. MicroRNAs are small (19–23-nt in length) non-coding regulatory RNAs that regulate the stability and/or translation of their target transcripts. MicroRNAs have been progressively implicated in all aspects of cell biology and homeostasis and established as key players in a number of pathologies, including, but not limited to, inflammatory, metabolic and cardiovascular diseases, neuropathologies, and cancers [14–26].

2. Resveratrol-Inducible *MiR-663* in Health and Disease

MicroRNAs that regulate fundamental functions, such as metabolism, cell proliferation and differentiation, or development, have generally been very well conserved between invertebrates and vertebrates during evolution. In contrast, other microRNAs are found in vertebrates only: thus, *miR-155*, a microRNA that has been implicated in inflammatory response and inflammation-associated cancers. Finally, some microRNAs are only found in one or a few species of vertebrates. This is the case for *miR-663* (a.k.a. *miR-663a*) that appears to be primate-specific. A few years ago, it was shown that, upon RSV treatment, *miR-663* was upregulated both in human THP-1 monocytes, where it targets transcripts encoding pro-inflammatory JunB and JunD, and in human SW480 colon cancer cells, where it targets *TGFβ1* transcripts [27,28] (Table 1). At first, this suggested that this microRNA by and large would deliver beneficial effects to the body. Nevertheless, available literature shows that this is not always the case (see here after), indicating that *miR-663* can be harmful as well, depending on the cellular context.

2.1. MiR-663 in Inflammation

The capability of RSV to modulate a wide range of signaling pathways implicated in both the mounting and the termination of the immune response have puzzled scientists for a long time. It is becoming increasingly clear that many of these effects of RSV are through the modification of the composition of microRNA populations within the cell [13,29]. Namely, microRNAs are global regulators with the capability to directly regulate tens to hundreds of target transcripts, and many more through indirect regulation that results from microRNAs targeting transcripts encoding regulators such as transcription factors, factors implicated in different signal transduction pathways, such as kinases or phosphatases, or epigenetic regulators such as methylases or demethylases.

For example, *miR-663* has been shown to decrease AP-1 activity, that is critical for the mounting of the inflammatory response, by directly targeting *JunB* and *JunD* transcripts, at least in part through the downregulation of *miR-155* [27]. In addition, RSV impairs the up-regulation of pro-inflammatory *miR-155* at least in part through increasing *miR-663* expression [27]. This property of RSV is likely to have major consequences, for *miR-155* is implicated in the mounting of both the innate and adaptive immune responses [16,30]. A study conducted on 35 hypertensive patients with coronary artery disease and type 2 diabetes showed that, after ingesting a grape extract containing RSV for one year, patients presented with peripheral blood mononuclear cells that expressed less pro-inflammatory IL-1β and TNFα cytokines, less pro-inflammatory *miR-155*, and more anti-inflammatory *miR-663*. Although conducted on a relatively small sample of patients, this study provides a good evidence that long lasting, low RSV doses have actual beneficial effects on patient health [31]. Incidentally, it further suggests that RSV might be a better candidate for preventive rather than for curative therapeutics, at least when it comes to inflammation-related pathologies.

In contrast, in patients with systemic lupus erythematous, *miR-663* impairs the proliferation and migration of bone marrow-derived mesenchymal stem cells, thus shifting the imbalance between follicular T helper cells and regulatory T cells toward less regulatory T cells and more follicular T helper cells. As regulatory T cells reduce the capability of B cells to augment autoimmunity, *miR-663* activity, by reducing the secretion of *TGFβ1* by T cells, worsens lupus development [32]. In addition, *miR-663* activity proved deleterious in rheumatoid arthritis, a disease linked to synovial inflammation, cartilage erosion and joint destruction. In fibroblast-like synoviocytes from rheumatoid arthritis patients, increased levels of *miR-663* suppressed the expression of *Adenomatous polyposis coli* (*APC*) gene, triggering the activation of the canonical Wnt signaling pathway through accumulation of β-catenin. This activation increases the production of pro-inflammatory cytokines and, as a consequence of increased inflammation in joints, disturb the osteoblast–osteoclast axis and increases bone resorption by osteoclasts [33].

Nuclear factor TDP-43 (trans-activation response element DNA-binding protein 43) is an RNA-binding protein that shuttles between the nucleus and the cytoplasm. TDP-43 in particular plays a role in the biogenesis of microRNAs through its interactions with the nuclear Drosha complex, which generates pre-miRNAs from pri-miRNAs, and the cytoplasmic Dicer complex, which then produces mature miRNAs from pre-miRNAs [34]. TDP-43 has been shown to be causative in amyotrophic lateral sclerosis (ALS) and frontotemporal dementia (FTD) [35]. Interestingly, TDP-43 can bind microRNAs such as *let-7b* and *miR-663*. TDP-43 knockdown in cultured cells decreases *let-7b* levels while increasing that of *miR-663*, thus modulating their activities [36]. It is thus possible that the role played by TDP-43 in neurodegenerative pathologies might be linked to its differential effects on microRNA production, and ultimately depends on whether these microRNAs are beneficial or deleterious in the context.

Finally, radiation-induced bystander effect corresponds to the biological response to radiations of cells that, while not being located in the path of ionizing rays, receive signals produced by directly irradiated cells that lead them to amplify or exaggerate the action of low dose radiation. This effect can significantly increase radiation risk and tissue damage. In particular, *TGFβ1* secretion by directly irradiated Hela cells reduces the expression of *miR-663* in both directly irradiated and bystander Hela cells, which correlates with increased DNA damage and reduced rate of cell survival. At the same time, *TGFβ1* signaling increases the expression of *miR-663* in bystander cells, which in turn decreases the levels of *TGFβ1* by targeting *TGFβ1* transcripts. By reducing *TGFβ1*-induced DNA damage, *miR-663* increases the survival of bystander cells, thus limiting the propagation of radiation-induced bystander effects [37]. Hence, the study of the effects of a low irradiation dose provides a further evidence for *miR-663* activity being at the same time beneficial as well as deleterious.

Therefore, the functions of *miR-663* seem to be context-dependent: it may well be that, in a given setting, the outcome of *miR-663* activity might depend on the context, i.e., on the transcriptome expressed in a given cell, and especially the panel of *miR-663* target transcripts that are present. It is also most probable that *miR-663* effects might be dose-dependent, and that it might target different transcripts as it has previously been shown for several microRNAs. For example, *miR-155* targeting of *Quaking* transcripts in RAW264.7 macrophages occurred at low concentration only [38], and, in myeloid cell from patients with acute myeloid leukemia, *miR-155* activity increases and decreases the levels of different set of transcripts depending of the level of *miR-155* expression [39]. Of note, RSV has the capability to change the level of expression of both *miR-155* and *miR-663* microRNAs, in both cases with apparent beneficial outcome [26,27]. Many other pathologies have also been associated with high levels of *miR-155*. For example, this microRNA has recently been shown to be causative in paralysis that develops following thoracic abdominal aortic aneurysm repair [40]. On the other hand, increased expression of chromosome 21-located *miR-155* in the brain of individuals with Down's dementia has been linked with the presence of hyperphosphorylated tau protein and the reduction of the levels of several *miR-155* targets, including BACH1, CoREST1, BCL6, BIM, BCL10, Cyclin D, and SAPK4 [41]. Therefore, the capability of *miR-663* to decrease *miR-155* expression [29] and reported capability of RSV to cerebral ischemia, in particular through its anti-inflammatory effects, [9] suggests that this compound might be protective when administered ahead of programmed surgery or intervention.

2.2. MiR-663 in Cancer

It is now recognized that microRNAs play a central role in molecular dysfunctions linking inflammation with cancer [42,43]. While certain microRNAs are generally considered as pro-oncogenic or oncomiRs and others as tumor-suppressors, it seems that their actual impact on cancers might be context- and/or dose-dependent. This is in particular the case for *miR-155*, that is implicated in the mounting of a robust anti-tumor immunity when expressed at high doses but favors tumorigenesis when expressed at moderate level [39,42,43]. More generally, changes in microRNA expression either are causative in the initiation of cancers, or a consequence of the process of tumorigenesis itself. Remarkably, *miR-155* displays mutator activity, in particular due to its targeting of transcripts encoding the cell-cycle regulator WEE1 [44].

As seen here above for inflammation, *miR-663* can either inhibit or favor cell proliferation and/or migration in different settings. In human MCF7 breast cancer cells, *miR-663* targets transcripts encoding Eukaryotic translation elongation factor 1A2 (eEF1A2), which results in slowing the proliferation of MCF7 cells. RSV treatment of these cells increased the expression of *miR-663* and *miR-744*, with a similar output [45]. Breast cancer has a higher incidence in young Lebanese women as compared with American woman. A comparative profiling study showed that, in Lebanese breast cancer patients, 21 miRNAs, including *miR-663*, were specifically deregulated, possibly as a result of differential methylation of their promoter [46]. Another study showed that *miR-663* is up-regulated in multidrug-resistant MDA-MB-231-derived ADM cell line, and that increased *miR-663* expression was associated with the downregulation of Heparin sulfate proteoglycan 2 (HSPG2) and chemoresistance [47].

MiR-663 was also shown to increase the proliferation of nasopharyngeal carcinoma NPC C666-1 cells by directly targeting the cell cycle negative regulator CDKN2A [48]. Accordingly, *miR-663* expression was higher in the serum of nasopharyngeal carcinoma patients, as compared with controls, and increasing *miR-663* levels were correlated with malignant progression and poor prognosis. On the other hand, *miR-663* expression was decreased by chemoradiotherapy [49]. The oncogenic activity of *miR-663* in nasopharyngeal carcinoma was due to its targeting of p21(WAF1/CIP1) that promotes the cellular G1/S transition [50]. In contrast, in two papillary thyroid carcinoma cell lines, *miR-663* behaved as a tumor-suppressor by targeting *TGFβ1*, thus inhibiting epithelium-to-mesenchyme transition [51], similar to what was previously found in SW480 colon cancer cells [28]. Similarly, *miR-663* levels were low in several human gastric cancer cell lines, and transfecting the two human gastric cancer cell lines

BGC823 and SNU5 with *miR-663* suppressed their proliferation and induced a phenotype of mitotic catastrophe, indicating that *miR-663* behaves as a tumor-suppressor in this type of cancer [52]. A study about the effects of sunitinib treatment of metastatic renal cell carcinoma patients showed that the resistance that these patients develop eventually is linked to the downregulation of *miR-1* and *miR-663*. This downregulation was associated with the acquisition of a migratory phenotype, as established on xenografts. In sunitinib resistant tumor cells, *miR-663* targets *FRAS1* (Fraser Extracellular Matrix Complex Subunit 1) and *MDGA1* (MAM Domain Containing Glycosylphosphatidylinositol Anchor 1) transcripts. Restoring *miR-1* and *miR-663* levels or knocking down MDGA1 decreased renal cancer cell proliferation and migration [53]. The expression of *miR-663* was upregulated in HepG2 hepatocellular carcinoma cells co-incubated with the endoplasmic reticulum stress inducer tunicamycin. In these cells, *miR-663* inhibited apoptosis induced by endoplasmic reticulum stress by targeting *TGFβ1* transcripts [54]. In agreement with this result, *miR-663* was one of seven microRNAs whose expression was specifically changed in patients with hepatitis B virus-related HCC [55]. In pancreatic cancer tissues and cell lines, the downregulation of *miR-663* inversely correlated with the upregulation of transcripts encoding eEF1A2. eEF1A2 and *miR-663* levels were linked with TNM (tumor/node/metastasis) stage and node metastasis status in the patients. *MiR-663* was shown to decrease the proliferation and invasion potentials of pancreatic cancer cells both in vitro and in vivo by directly targeting *eEF1A2* [56]. A study about colorectal cancer, based on 109 biopsy specimens, compared biopsied from patients with tubulovillous adenomas and high-grade dysplasia versus biopsies from patients with normal mucosa or hyperplastic polyps. It showed that, among 99 microRNAs whose expression was different between the two groups, *miR-663*, *miR-1268*, *miR-320b*, *miR-1275*, and *miR-320b* were the most upregulated microRNAs in the biopsies of the first group of patients [49]. *MiR-663* was also upregulated in biopsies from cutaneous tissues with malignant melanoma [57].

Patients with lung cancers present with high level of *miR-663* expression, and *miR-663* direct or indirect targeting of *TGFβ1*, *P53*, *Bax*, and *Fas* transcripts increased the proliferation of A549 lung cancer cells [58]. Accordingly, *miR-663* proved deleterious in non-small cell lung cancer cells by targeting *PUMA/BBC3* (p53 up-regulated modulator of apoptosis/Bcl-2 binding component 3) and *BTG2* (B-cell translocation gene 2) transcripts, thus allowing cancer cells to escape apoptosis and promoting tumor onset and development [59]. Nevertheless, waltonitone treatment inhibited proliferation and induced apoptosis of H460 and H3255 lung cancer cell lines at least in part through inducing the targeting of *Bcl-2* by *miR-663* [60]. These results provide a further illustration of the ambiguous role *miR-663* can play in a particular type of tumor.

In a study on glioblastomas, the most aggressive brain tumor, the grade of tumors correlated with the level of PI3KCD activity (phosphatidylinositol-4,5-bisphosphate 3 kinase catalytic subunit delta) but inversely correlated with the level of *miR-663* expression. Higher *miR-663* levels were associated with increased patient survival, which was linked with *miR-663* targeting transcripts encoding PI3KCD [61]. *MiR-663* was also shown to decrease glioblastoma by targeting transcripts encoding CXCR4, the receptor of chemokine CXCL12 that is known to be involved in glioblastoma progression, and *miR-663* overexpression prolonged survival of mice with glioblastoma [62]. *MiR-663* was downregulated in A172 and U87 glioblastoma cell lines. Transfecting these cells with *miR-663* inhibited their proliferation, migration and invasion. These effects were through *miR-663* direct targeting of *TGFβ1*, as well as transcripts encoding *TGFβ1* downstream mediators MMP2 (Matrix metalloprotease 2) and E-cadherin [63]. On the other hand, *miR-663* expression was upregulated in castration-resistant prostate cancer tissues, and *miR-663* overexpression in LNCaP prostate cancer cells increased their potentials for proliferation, invasion and neuroendocrine differentiation, while reducing dihydrotestosterone-induced upregulation of prostate-specific antigen expression. In situ hybridization experiments established that the level of expression of *miR-663* correlates with TNM stage and Gleason score and is a good predictor of cancer recurrence [64]. In a meta-analysis, STAT3 (Signal Transducers and Activators of Transcription 3), JUN and JUNB transcription factors were identified as key signatures of a metastatic integrative regulatory network in prostate cancer progression. *MiR-663*, that is overexpressed in these types of cancers, was one of five microRNAs responsible for the down-regulation of the genes encoding these three transcription factors [65]. *MiR-663*, along with *miR-622* and *miR-647*, was upregulated in Taxol-resistant ovarian cancer cells, and the survival of Taxol-resistant patients with lower levels of *miR-663* and *miR-622* expression was significantly longer than patients with higher levels of expression of these two microRNAs [66].

As for liquid malignancies, *miR-663* was downregulated in K-562 cell line and in the white blood cells of certain patients with chronic myelogenous leukemia, due to the aberrant methylation of CpG islands upstream of *miR-663* gene. *MiR-663* suppressed K-562 cell proliferation at least in part through the targeting of *H-ras* transcripts [67]. The promoter of *miR-663* was also found to be hypermethylated in Chinese pediatric acute myeloid leukemia [68]. *MiR-663* was one of nine microRNAs most constantly upregulated in multiple myeloma cell lines. The upregulation of these microRNAs, including *miR-663* and *miR-155*, was linked with decreased viability, migration and colony formation of these cell lines. In addition, the higher expression levels of these microRNAs correlated with better patient survival [69]. Thus, *miR-663* behaves as a tumor-suppressor in liquid malignancies, in agreement with previous results showing that *all-trans* retinoic acid, a powerful pro-differentiation agent, induces the differentiation of HL-60 acute myeloid leukemia cells through the up-regulation of *miR-663* [70].

Epigenetic deregulation of *miR-663* expression appears to be a rather general feature of liquid malignancies. Of note, it was recently shown that the regulation of *miR-663* expression through epigenetic modification of its promoter depends of mitochondria-to-nucleus retrograde signaling, as shown by the downregulation of *miR-663* in cells lacking mitochondria, and also that *miR-663* mediates mitochondria-to-nucleus retrograde signaling [71]. Mitochondrial impairment through pharmacological disruption of oxidative phosphorylations, that increases reactive oxygen species, reduces *miR-663* expression. *MiR-663* regulates the expression of nuclear-encoded respiratory chain subunits involved in Complexes I, II, III, and IV, as well as that of Complexes I (NDUFAF1), II (SDHAF2), III (UQCC2), and IV (SCO1) assembly factor. In particular, *miR-663* activity is required for stabilizing respiratory supercomplexes, and directly regulated *UQCC2* expression. Mitochondrial dysfunction is one of the hallmarks of cancer, and indeed *miR-663* ectopic expression decreased tumor weight in xenografts and decreased cellular invasiveness of MCF7 and MDA-MB-231 breast cancer cell lines [71].

In conclusion, *miR-663* can either promote or inhibit tumorigenesis and metastasis depending on the context and the type of tumors. It remains to be shown whether it could be possible to turn *miR-663* from deleterious to beneficial in tumors where its activity correlates with increased tumorigenesis, rather than trying to inhibit its expression. RSV could be a good candidate compound, given its established anti-proliferation and anti-tumors effects associated with it capability to modulate the expression of *miR-663* along with that of other microRNAs. Of note, RSV effects in different cancers may have epigenetic bases, given its capacity to modulate the expression of NAD^+-dependent histone deacetylases (Sirtuins), and particularly to activate Sirt1 and Sirt5 while inhibiting Sirt3 activity [72].

2.3. MiR-663 in Atherosclerosis

Atherosclerosis is a chronic inflammatory disease of the vascular wall, which, if left unchecked, turns into pathologies such as myocardial infarction and ischemic stroke, that are some the most prevalent causes of morbidity and lethality in the most developed countries. Atherosclerosis, although associated with systemic risk factors such as hypercholesterolemia, hypertension, and diabetes mellitus, most usually initiates in regions exposed to disturbed blood flow (d-flow), while arterial regions exposed to stable flow (s-flow) remain healthy [73]. It has been established that d-flow induces, and s-flow prevents endothelial dysfunction and atherosclerosis, respectively, at least in part through alterations in gene expression associated with changes in the epigenetic landscape [73]. Among these genes, microRNAs have been classified into three categories depending on their effects on atherogenesis: antiatherogenic mechano-miRs, proatherogenic mechano-miRs, and dual-role mechano-miRs [73].

MiR-663 was identified among microRNAs that were upregulated in umbilical vein endothelial cells (HUVECs) submitted to oscillatory shear stress. In these cells, *miR-663* was implicated in monocyte adhesion but not in apoptosis [74]. It was subsequently shown that, in endothelial cells, *miR-663* plays a role in the upregulation of the gene encoding the transcription factor ATF4 and of its downstream gene VEGF, as well as in the activation of the ATF4 branch of unfolded protein response by oxidized phospholipids [75]. It was further shown that high concentrations of uric acid inhibit endothelial cell migration by upregulating *miR-663*, that directly targets *TGFβ1*. Higher *miR-663* levels were also found in the serum of hyperuricemic patients and animals [76]. Nevertheless, *miR-663* was shown to inhibit vascular smooth muscular cell phenotypic switch (the transformation from a contractile, differentiate phenotype to a synthetic, dedifferentiated phenotype associated with artery injury) by targeting *JUNB* and *MYH9* (myosin light chain 9 expression) transcripts [77]. *MiR-663* was further implicated in the induction of atherosclerosis by *Helicobacter pylori* [78].

Table 1. Validated and putative target transcripts of *miR-663* that link this microRNA with inflammatory, neurodegenerative and cardiovascular diseases, as well as with cancer.

Target Transcripts	MiR-663 Effects	References
	Opposite effects on inflammation	
JunB, JunD	Anti-inflammatory, through reducing AP-1 activity and *miR-155* expression	[27]
TGFβ1	Worsens lupus erythematous development	[32]
APC	Pro-inflammatory through the activation of Wnt pathway	[33]
	Stimulation of cell proliferation and migration	
TGFβ1	Increases the survival of non-irradiated bystander cells	[37]
HSPG2	Increases chemoresistance of MDA-MB-231/ADM cell line	[47]
TGFβ1	Inhibits apoptosis induced by endoplasmic reticulum stress	[54]
TGFβ1, P53, Bax, Fas	Increases lung cancer cell proliferation	[57]
PUMA/BBC3, BTG2	Inhibits apoptosis and promotes tumor development	[59]
	Inhibition of cell proliferation and migration	
eEF1A2	Impairs the proliferation of MCF7 cells	[45]
CDKN2A	Promotes the proliferation of nasopharyngeal carcinoma C666-1 cells	[48]
p21(WAF1/CIP1)	Promotes the proliferation of nasopharyngeal carcinoma cells	[50]
TGFβ1	Antimetastatic in SW480 colorectal cancer cells	[28]
TGFβ1	Inhibits epithelium-to-mesenchyme transition of two thyroid carcinoma cell lines	[51]
MDGA1, FRAS1	decreases renal cancer cell proliferation and migration	[53]
eEF1A2	Inhibits proliferation and invasion of pancreatic cancer cells	[56]
Bcl-2	Implicated in waltonitone treatment-induced inhibition of lung cancer cell line proliferation	[60]
PI3KCD	Inhibits proliferation and invasiveness of glioblastoma cells	[61]
CXCR4	Increases survival of mice with glioblastoma	[62]
TGFβ1, MMP2, E-Cadherin	Inhibits proliferation and invasiveness of glioblastoma cells	[63]
H-ras	Inhibits proliferation of K-562 cells	[67]
UQCC2	Increases phosphorylative oxidations and decreases tumor development	[72]
	Prevention of arterial injury	
TGFβ1	Inhibits endothelial cell migration under high concentrations of uric acid	[76]
JUNB, MYH9	Inhibits vascular smooth muscular cell phenotypic switch	[77]

Finally, as previously mentioned, a study conducted on peripheral blood mononuclear cells of type 2 diabetes and hypertensive patients with coronary showed that one-year supplementation with a grape extract containing RSV modulates the expression of inflammation-related microRNAs and cytokines expression [31]. In particular, pro-inflammatory *miR-155* was down-regulated, while *miR-663* was up-regulated, with correlative downregulation of *JUND* [31], a validated target of *miR-663* [27].

3. Conclusions

The literature analyzed here above clearly demonstrates that it goes for microRNAs as it goes for coding genes: none of them is just only detrimental, none of them is capable of producing beneficial effects in all circumstances. Thus, the analysis of molecular effects and functions of this class of regulators requires a rather expressionist approach, looking for bright effects aside the deleterious ones. This is in particular the case for *miR-663*, that, as seen in Table 1, depending on the context and the type of cells and tumors considered, can be either pro- or anti-inflammatory, or behave either as a tumor-suppressor gene or well favor tumorigenesis. Also, while *miR-663* has been several times described as a "bad" microRNA, it nevertheless seems capable to deliver tumor-suppressive effects and to prevent vascular smooth muscular cell phenotypic switch that is associated with arterial injury.

Although microRNAs can successively, or possibly at the same time, behave as the bad, the good or the ugly, like the heroes of the classical Western movie with a similar name, one impressive conclusion that can be drawn from the study of the effects of RSV on *miR-663* expression is that this biological compound has the remarkable propriety to induce the good behavior while inhibiting the bad and the ugly ones. Thus, it has been previously shown that RSV treatment of SW480 colon cancer cells leads to both the downregulation of microRNAs known to favor cancer initiation and progression and the upregulation of microRNAs usually considered as tumor-suppressors, including *miR-663* in this context [28]. In this respect, it should be noted that both, *miR-663* and RSV are implicated in the regulation of the *TGFβ1* signaling pathway. This might possibly explain at least in part why RSV can deliver beneficial effects trough the modulation of *miR-663* expression, given that *TGFβ1* can be cytostatic at the early stages of cancer while also favoring epithelium-to-mesenchyme transition at more advances stages of tumorization, owing to the similar function it plays during development. In addition, *TGFβ1* is also implicated in the regulation of the immune response, and systemic immune suppression and inhibition of host immunosurveillance favors cancer development [79]. Furthermore, it has been shown that *TGFβ1* up-regulates *miR-155* in hepatocellular carcinoma cells, thus promoting epithelium-to-mesenchyme transition, invasion and metastasis [80], and that *miR-155* plays a role in mediating *TGFβ1*-induced podocyte injury via nephrin, desmin and caspase-9 [81]. Therefore, the capability of RSV to modulate, directly or indirectly, the levels of *miR-155*, *miR-663* and *TGFβ1* activity, and the fact that the three last molecules display dose-dependent activity and can be either beneficial or deleterious to the body, depending on the context, may possibly explain the apparent pleiotropic beneficial effects of RSV, and certainly warrants further studies.

Given that RSV seems to be active while provided at low dose for a sustained period, rather than at higher doses for a shorter period, it is possible that the wide range of beneficial properties of this plant polyphenol may rely on its capacity to simultaneously reset the expression of multiple microRNAs within a range of concentrations where they would work for the health of the organism, rather than just sharply increasing or decreasing their expression. This might possibly explain RSV apparent lack of delivering increasingly beneficial effects at increasing doses, a fact that led to suggest that most of RSV apparent properties may rather result from experimental artifacts. Beside all its proved or potential beneficial effects to the health of the individual, RSV may well provide us with a new tool for the study of dose-dependent activity of microRNAs and other non-coding regulatory RNAs in the future.

Author Contributions: J.-J.M., V.P., B.R., H.K., E.C.F., and E.T. participated equally in the analysis of the literature data. J.-J.M. and E.T. organized and wrote the manuscript.

Funding: This research received no external funding. Page: 8.

Conflicts of Interest: The authors declare no conflict of interest.

References

1. Delmas, D.; Lançon, A.; Colin, D.; Jannin, B.; Latruffe, N. Resveratrol as a chemopreventive agent: A promising molecule for fighting cancer. *Curr. Drug Targets* **2006**, *7*, 423–442. [CrossRef] [PubMed]
2. Tili, E.; Michaille, J.-J. Resveratrol, MicroRNAs, Inflammation, and Cancer. *J. Nucleic Acids* **2011**, *2011*, 102431. [CrossRef] [PubMed]
3. Sinha, D.; Sarkar, N.; Biswas, J.; Bishayee, A. Resveratrol for breast cancer prevention and therapy: Preclinical evidence and molecular mechanisms. *Semin. Cancer Biol.* **2016**, *40–41*, 209–232. [CrossRef] [PubMed]
4. Bartolacci, C.; Andreani, C.; Amici, A.; Marchini, C. Walking a Tightrope: A Perspective of Resveratrol Effects on Breast Cancer. *Curr. Protein Pept. Sci.* **2018**, *19*, 311–322. [CrossRef] [PubMed]

5. Zordoky, B.N.; Robertson, I.M.; Dyck, J.R. Preclinical and clinical evidence for the role of resveratrol in the treatment of cardiovascular diseases. *Biochim. Biophys. Acta* **2015**, *1852*, 1155–1177. [CrossRef] [PubMed]
6. Erdogan, C.S.; Vang, O. Challenges in analyzing the biological effects of resveratrol. *Nutrients* **2016**, *8*, 353. [CrossRef] [PubMed]
7. Singh, C.K.; Ndiaye, M.A.; Ahmad, N. Resveratrol and cancer: Challenges for clinical translation. *Biochim. Biophys. Acta* **2015**, *1852*, 1178–1185. [CrossRef] [PubMed]
8. Ko, J.H.; Sethi, G.; Um, J.Y.; Shanmugam, M.K.; Arfuso, F.; Kumar, A.P.; Bishayee, A.; Ahn, K.S. The Role of Resveratrol in Cancer Therapy. *Int. J. Mol. Sci.* **2017**, *18*, 2589. [CrossRef] [PubMed]
9. Lee, R.H.C.; Lee, M.H.H.; Wu, C.Y.C.; Couto e Silva, A.; Possoit, H.E.; Hsieh, T.H.; Minagar, A.; Lin, H.W. Cerebral ischemia and neuroregeneration. *Neural Regen. Res.* **2018**, *13*, 373–385. [CrossRef] [PubMed]
10. Rauf, A.; Imran, M.; Suleria, H.A.R.; Ahmad, B.; Peters, D.G.; Mubarak, M.S. A comprehensive review of the health perspectives of resveratrol. *Food Funct.* **2017**, *8*, 4284–4305. [CrossRef] [PubMed]
11. Bonnefont-Rousselot, D. Resveratrol and Cardiovascular Diseases. *Nutrients* **2016**, *8*, 250. [CrossRef] [PubMed]
12. Fogacci, F.; Tocci, G.; Presta, V.; Fratter, A.; Borghi, C.; Cicero, A.F.G. Effect of resveratrol on blood pressure: A systematic review and meta-analysis of randomized, controlled, clinical trials. *Crit. Rev. Food Sci. Nutr.* **2018**, *23*, 1–14. [CrossRef] [PubMed]
13. Tili, E.; Michaille, J.-J. Promiscuous Effects of Some Phenolic Natural Products on Inflammation at Least in Part Arise from Their Ability to Modulate the Expression of Global Regulators, Namely microRNAs. *Molecules* **2016**, *21*, 1263. [CrossRef] [PubMed]
14. Neudecker, V.; Yuan, X.; Bowser, J.L.; Eltzschig, H.K. MicroRNAs in mucosal inflammation. *J. Mol. Med.* **2017**, *95*, 935–949. [CrossRef] [PubMed]
15. Tili, E.; Michaille, J.-J.; Piurowski, V.; Rigot, B.; Croce, C.M. MicroRNAs in intestinal barrier function, inflammatory bowel disease and related cancers-their effects and therapeutic potentials. *Curr. Opin. Pharmacol.* **2017**, *37*, 142–150. [CrossRef] [PubMed]
16. Alivernini, S.; Gremese, E.; McSharry, C.; Tolusso, B.; Ferraccioli, G.; McInnes, I.B.; Kurowska-Stolarska, M. MicroRNA-155-at the Critical Interface of Innate and Adaptive Immunity in Arthritis. *Front. Immunol.* **2018**, *8*, 1932. [CrossRef] [PubMed]
17. Momen-Heravi, F.; Bala, S. miRNA regulation of innate immunity. *J. Leukoc. Biol.* **2018**. [CrossRef] [PubMed]
18. Curtale, G. MiRNAs at the Crossroads between Innate Immunity and Cancer: Focus on Macrophages. *Cells* **2018**, *7*, 12. [CrossRef] [PubMed]
19. Mirra, P.; Nigro, C.; Prevenzano, I.; Leone, A.; Raciti, G.A.; Formisano, P.; Beguinot, F.; Miele, C. The Destiny of Glucose from a MicroRNA Perspective. *Front. Endocrinol.* **2018**, *9*, 46. [CrossRef] [PubMed]
20. Wojciechowska, A.; Braniewska, A.; Kozar-Kamińska, K. MicroRNA in cardiovascular biology and disease. *Adv. Clin. Exp. Med.* **2017**, *26*, 865–874. [CrossRef] [PubMed]
21. Vogiatzi, G.; Oikonomou, E.; Deftereos, S.; Siasos, G.; Tousoulis, D. Peripheral artery disease: A micro-RNA-related condition? *Curr. Opin. Pharmacol.* **2018**, *39*, 105–112. [CrossRef] [PubMed]
22. Miya Shaik, M.; Tamargo, I.A.; Abubakar, M.B.; Kamal, M.A.; Greig, N.H.; Gan, S.H. The Role of microRNAs in Alzheimer's Disease and Their Therapeutic Potentials. *Genes* **2018**, *9*, 174. [CrossRef] [PubMed]
23. Narayan, N.; Bracken, C.P.; Ekert, P.G. MicroRNA-155 expression and function in AML: An evolving paradigm. *Exp. Hematol.* **2018**, *27*, 30165–30166. [CrossRef] [PubMed]
24. Farooqi, A.A.; Khalid, S.; Ahmad, A. Regulation of Cell Signaling Pathways and miRNAs by Resveratrol in Different Cancers. *Int. J. Mol. Sci.* **2018**, *19*, 652. [CrossRef] [PubMed]
25. Vannini, I.; Fanini, F.; Fabbri, M. Emerging roles of microRNAs in cancer. *Curr. Opin. Genet. Dev.* **2018**, *48*, 128–133. [CrossRef] [PubMed]
26. Ramassone, A.; Pagotto, S.; Veronese, A.; Visone, R. Epigenetics and MicroRNAs in Cancer. *Int. J. Mol. Sci.* **2018**, *19*, 459. [CrossRef] [PubMed]
27. Tili, E.; Michaille, J.-J.; Adair, B.; Alder, H.; Limagne, E.; Taccioli, C.; Ferracin, M.; Delmas, D.; Latruffe, N.; Croce, C.M. Resveratrol decreases the levels of miR-155 by upregulating miR-663, a microRNA targeting JunB and JunD. *Carcinogenesis* **2010**, *31*, 1561–1566. [CrossRef] [PubMed]

28. Tili, E.; Michaille, J.-J.; Alder, H.; Volinia, S.; Delmas, D.; Latruffe, N.; Croce, C.M. Resveratrol modulates the levels of microRNAs targeting genes encoding tumor-suppressors and effectors of *TGFβ* signaling pathway in SW480 cells. *Biochem. Pharmacol.* **2010**, *80*, 2057–2065. [CrossRef] [PubMed]
29. Latruffe, N.; Lançon, A.; Frazzi, R.; Aires, V.; Delmas, D.; Michaille, J.-J.; Djouadi, F.; Bastin, J.; Cherkaoui-Malki, M. Exploring new ways of regulation by resveratrol involving miRNAs, with emphasis on inflammation. *Ann. N. Y. Acad. Sci.* **2015**, *1348*, 97–106. [CrossRef] [PubMed]
30. Tili, E.; Michaille, J.-J.; Cimino, A.; Costinean, S.; Dumitru, C.D.; Adair, B.; Fabbri, M.; Alder, H.; Liu, C.G.; Calin, G.A.; et al. Modulation of miR-155 and miR-125b levels following lipopolysaccharide/TNF-alpha stimulation and their possible roles in regulating the response to endotoxin shock. *J. Immunol.* **2007**, *179*, 5082–5089. [CrossRef] [PubMed]
31. Tomé-Carneiro, J.; Larrosa, M.; Yáñez-Gascón, M.J.; Dávalos, A.; Gil-Zamorano, J.; Gonzálvez, M.; García-Almagro, F.J.; Ruiz Ros, J.A.; Tomás-Barberán, F.A.; Espín, J.C.; et al. One-year supplementation with a grape extract containing resveratrol modulates inflammatory-related microRNAs and cytokines expression in peripheral blood mononuclear cells of type 2 diabetes and hypertensive patients with coronary artery disease. *Pharmacol. Res.* **2013**, *72*, 69–82. [CrossRef] [PubMed]
32. Geng, L.; Tang, X.; Zhou, K.; Wang, D.; Wang, S.; Yao, G.; Chen, W.; Gao, X.; Chen, W.; Shi, S.; et al. MicroRNA-663 induces immune dysregulation by inhibiting *TGF-β1* production in bone marrow-derived mesenchymal stem cells in patients with systemic lupus erythematosus. *Cell. Mol. Immunol.* **2018**. [CrossRef] [PubMed]
33. Miao, C.G.; Shi, W.J.; Xiong, Y.Y.; Yu, H.; Zhang, X.L.; Qin, M.S.; Du, C.L.; Song, T.W.; Zhang, B.; Li, J. MicroRNA-663 activates the canonical Wnt signaling through the adenomatous polyposis coli suppression. *Immunol. Lett.* **2015**, *166*, 45–54. [CrossRef] [PubMed]
34. Kawahara, Y.; Mieda-Sato, A. TDP-43 promotes microRNA biogenesis as a component of the Drosha and Dicer complexes. *Proc. Natl. Acad. Sci. USA* **2012**, *109*, 3347–3352. [CrossRef] [PubMed]
35. Ling, S.C.; Polymenidou, M.; Cleveland, D.W. Converging mechanisms in ALS and FTD: Disrupted RNA and protein homeostasis. *Neuron* **2013**, *79*, 416–438. [CrossRef] [PubMed]
36. Buratti, E.; De Conti, L.; Stuani, C.; Romano, M.; Baralle, M.; Baralle, F. Nuclear factor TDP-43 can affect selected microRNA levels. *FEBS J.* **2010**, *277*, 2268–2281. [CrossRef] [PubMed]
37. Hu, W.; Xu, S.; Yao, B.; Hong, M.; Wu, X.; Pei, H.; Chang, L.; Ding, N.; Gao, X.; Ye, C.; et al. MiR-663 inhibits radiation-induced bystander effects by targeting *TGFβ1* in a feedback mode. *RNA Biol.* **2014**, *11*, 1189–1198. [CrossRef] [PubMed]
38. Tili, E.; Chiabai, M.; Palmieri, D.; Brown, M.; Cui, R.; Fernandes, C.; Richmond, T.; Kim, T.; Sheetz, T.; Sun, H.L.; et al. Quaking and miR-155 interactions in inflammation and leukemogenesis. *Oncotarget* **2015**, *6*, 24599–24610. [CrossRef] [PubMed]
39. Narayan, N.; Morenos, L.; Phipson, B.; Willis, S.N.; Brumatti, G.; Eggers, S.; Lalaoui, N.; Brown, L.M.; Kosasih, H.J.; Bartolo, R.C.; et al. Functionally distinct roles for different miR-155 expression levels through contrasting effects on gene expression, in acute myeloid leukaemia. *Leukemia* **2017**, *31*, 808–820. [CrossRef] [PubMed]
40. Awad, H.; Bratasz, A.; Nuovo, G.; Burry, R.; Meng, X.; Kelani, H.; Brown, M.; Ramadan, M.E.; Bouhliqah, L.; Popovich, P.G.; et al. MiR-155 deletion reduces ischemia-induced paralysis in a TAAA repair mouse model. *Ann. Diagn. Pathol.* **2018**, *36*, 12–20. [CrossRef] [PubMed]
41. Tili, E.; Mezache, L.; Michaille, J.-J.; Amann, V.; Williams, J.; Vandiver, P.; Quinonez, M.; Fadda, P.; Mikhail, A.; Nuovo, G. microRNA 155 up regulation in the CNS is strongly correlated to Down's syndrome dementia. *Ann. Diagn. Pathol.* **2018**, *34*, 103–109. [CrossRef] [PubMed]
42. Tili, E.; Michaille, J.-J.; Croce, C.M. miR-155: On the crosstalk between inflammation and cancer. *Int. Rev. Immunol.* **2009**, *28*, 264–284. [CrossRef] [PubMed]
43. Tili, E.; Michaille, J.-J.; Croce, C.M. MicroRNAs play a central role in molecular dysfunctions linking inflammation with cancer. *Immunol. Rev.* **2013**, *253*, 167–184. [CrossRef] [PubMed]
44. Tili, E.; Michaille, J.-J.; Wernicke, D.; Alder, H.; Costinean, S.; Volinia, S.; Croce, C.M. Mutator activity induced by microRNA-155 (miR-155) links inflammation and cancer. *Proc. Natl. Acad. Sci. USA* **2011**, *108*, 4908–4913. [CrossRef] [PubMed]

45. Vislovukh, A.; Kratassiouk, G.; Porto, E.; Gralievska, N.; Beldiman, C.; Pinna, G.; El'skaya, A.; Harel-Bellan, A.; Negrutskii, B.; Groisman, I. Proto-oncogenic isoform A2 of eukaryotic translation elongation factor eEF1 is a target of miR-663 and miR-744. *Br. J. Cancer* **2013**, *108*, 2304–2311. [CrossRef] [PubMed]
46. Nassar, F.J.; Talhouk, R.; Zgheib, N.K.; Tfayli, A.; El Sabban, M.; El Saghir, N.S.; Boulos, F.; Jabbour, M.N.; Chalala, C.; Boustany, R.M.; et al. microRNA Expression in Ethnic Specific Early Stage Breast Cancer: An Integration and Comparative Analysis. *Sci. Rep.* **2017**, *7*, 16829. [CrossRef] [PubMed]
47. Hu, H.; Li, S.; Cui, X.; Lv, X.; Jiao, Y.; Yu, F.; Yao, H.; Song, E.; Chen, Y.; Wang, M.; et al. The overexpression of hypomethylated miR-663 induces chemotherapy resistance in human breast cancer cells by targeting heparin sulfate proteoglycan 2 (HSPG2). *J. Biol. Chem.* **2013**, *288*, 10973–10985. [CrossRef] [PubMed]
48. Liang, S.; Zhang, N.; Deng, Y.; Chen, L.; Zhang, Y.; Zheng, Z.; Luo, W.; Lv, Z.; Li, S.; Xu, T. miR-663 promotes NPC cell proliferation by directly targeting CDKN2A. *Mol. Med. Rep.* **2017**, *16*, 4863–4870. [CrossRef] [PubMed]
49. Tsikitis, V.L.; Potter, A.; Mori, M.; Buckmeier, J.A.; Preece, C.R.; Harrington, C.A.; Bartley, A.N.; Bhattacharyya, A.K.; Hamilton, S.R.; Lance, M.P.; et al. MicroRNA Signatures of Colonic Polyps on Screening and Histology. *Cancer Prev. Res.* **2016**, *9*, 942–949. [CrossRef] [PubMed]
50. Yi, C.; Wang, Q.; Wang, L.; Huang, Y.; Li, L.; Liu, L.; Zhou, X.; Xie, G.; Kang, T.; Wang, H.; et al. MiR-663, a microRNA targeting p21(WAF1/CIP1), promotes the proliferation and tumorigenesis of nasopharyngeal carcinoma. *Oncogene* **2012**, *31*, 4421–4433. [CrossRef] [PubMed]
51. Wang, Z.; Zhang, H.; Zhang, P.; Dong, W.; He, L. MicroRNA-663 suppresses cell invasion and migration by targeting transforming growth factor beta 1 in papillary thyroid carcinoma. *Tumor Biol.* **2016**, *37*, 7633–7644. [CrossRef] [PubMed]
52. Pan, J.; Hu, H.; Zhou, Z.; Sun, L.; Peng, L.; Yu, L.; Sun, L.; Liu, J.; Yang, Z.; Ran, Y. Tumor-suppressive mir-663 gene induces mitotic catastrophe growth arrest in human gastric cancer cells. *Oncol. Rep.* **2010**, *24*, 105–112. [PubMed]
53. Butz, H.; Ding, Q.; Nofech-Mozes, R.; Lichner, Z.; Ni, H.; Yousef, G.M. Elucidating mechanisms of sunitinib resistance in renal cancer: An integrated pathological-molecular analysis. *Oncotarget* **2017**, *9*, 4661–4674. [CrossRef] [PubMed]
54. Huang, Y.; Liu, J.; Fan, L.; Wang, F.; Yu, H.; Wei, W.; Sun, G. miR-663 overexpression induced by endoplasmic reticulum stress modulates hepatocellular carcinoma cell apoptosis via transforming growth factor beta 1. *OncoTargets Ther.* **2016**, *9*, 1623–1633. [CrossRef] [PubMed]
55. Wang, G.; Dong, F.; Xu, Z.; Sharma, S.; Hu, X.; Chen, D.; Zhang, L.; Zhang, J.; Dong, Q. MicroRNA profile in HBV-induced infection and hepatocellular carcinoma. *BMC Cancer* **2017**, *17*, 805. [CrossRef] [PubMed]
56. Zang, W.; Wang, Y.; Wang, T.; Du, Y.; Chen, X.; Li, M.; Zhao, G. miR-663 attenuates tumor growth and invasiveness by targeting eEF1A2 in pancreatic cancer. *Mol. Cancer* **2015**, *14*, 37. [CrossRef] [PubMed]
57. Sand, M.; Skrygan, M.; Sand, D.; Georgas, D.; Gambichler, T.; Hahn, S.A.; Altmeyer, P.; Bechara, F.G. Comparative microarray analysis of microRNA expression profiles in primary cutaneous malignant melanoma, cutaneous malignant melanoma metastases, and benign melanocytic nevi. *Cell Tissue Res.* **2013**, *351*, 85–98. [CrossRef] [PubMed]
58. Liu, Z.Y.; Zhang, G.L.; Wang, M.M.; Xiong, Y.N.; Cui, H.Q. MicroRNA-663 targets TGFB1 and regulates lung cancer proliferation. *Asian Pac. J. Cancer Prev.* **2011**, *12*, 2819–2823. [PubMed]
59. Fiori, M.E.; Villanova, L.; Barbini, C.; De Angelis, M.L.; De Maria, R. miR-663 sustains NSCLC by inhibiting mitochondrial outer membrane permeabilization (MOMP) through PUMA/BBC3 and BTG2. *Cell Death Dis.* **2018**, *9*, 49. [CrossRef] [PubMed]
60. Zhang, Y.; Zhou, X.; Xu, X.; Zhang, M.; Wang, X.; Bai, X.; Li, H.; Kan, L.; Zhou, Y.; Niu, H.; et al. Waltonitone induces apoptosis through mir-663-induced Bcl-2 downregulation in non-small cell lung cancer. *Tumour Biol.* **2015**, *36*, 871–876. [CrossRef] [PubMed]
61. Shi, Y.; Chen, C.; Zhang, X.; Liu, Q.; Xu, J.L.; Zhang, H.R.; Yao, X.H.; Jiang, T.; He, Z.C.; Ren, Y.; et al. Primate-specific miR-663 functions as a tumor suppressor by targeting PIK3CD and predicts the prognosis of human glioblastoma. *Clin. Cancer Res.* **2014**, *20*, 1803–1813. [CrossRef] [PubMed]

62. Shi, Y.; Chen, C.; Yu, S.Z.; Liu, Q.; Rao, J.; Zhang, H.R.; Xiao, H.L.; Fu, T.W.; Long, H.; He, Z.C.; et al. miR-663 Suppresses Oncogenic Function of CXCR4 in Glioblastoma. *Clin. Cancer Res.* **2015**, *21*, 4004–4013. [CrossRef] [PubMed]
63. Li, Q.; Cheng, Q.; Chen, Z.; Peng, R.; Chen, R.; Ma, Z.; Wan, X.; Liu, J.; Meng, M.; Peng, Z.; et al. MicroRNA-663 inhibits the proliferation, migration and invasion of glioblastoma cells via targeting TGF-β1. *Oncol. Rep.* **2016**, *35*, 1125–1134. [CrossRef] [PubMed]
64. Jiao, L.; Deng, Z.; Xu, C.; Yu, Y.; Li, Y.; Yang, C.; Chen, J.; Liu, Z.; Huang, G.; Li, L.C.; et al. miR-663 induces castration-resistant prostate cancer transformation and predicts clinical recurrence. *J. Cell. Physiol.* **2014**, *229*, 834–844. [CrossRef] [PubMed]
65. Sadeghi, M.; Ranjbar, B.; Ganjalikhany, M.R.; Khan, F.M.; Schmitz, U.; Wolkenhauer, O.; Gupta, S.K. MicroRNA and Transcription Factor Gene Regulatory Network Analysis Reveals Key Regulatory Elements Associated with Prostate Cancer Progression. *PLoS ONE* **2016**, *11*, e0168760. [CrossRef] [PubMed]
66. Kim, Y.W.; Kim, E.Y.; Jeon, D.; Liu, J.L.; Kim, H.S.; Choi, J.W.; Ahn, W.S. Differential microRNA expression signatures and cell type-specific association with Taxol resistance in ovarian cancer cells. *Drug Des. Devel. Ther.* **2014**, *8*, 293–314. [CrossRef] [PubMed]
67. Yang, Y.; Wang, L.L.; Wang, H.X.; Guo, Z.K.; Gao, X.F.; Cen, J.; Li, Y.H.; Dou, L.P.; Yu, L. The epigenetically-regulated miR-663 targets H-ras in K-562 cells. *FEBS J.* **2013**, *280*, 5109–5117. [CrossRef] [PubMed]
68. Yan-Fang, T.; Jian, N.; Jun, L.; Na, W.; Pei-Fang, X.; Wen-Li, Z.; Dong, W.; Li, P.; Jian, W.; Xing, F.; et al. The promoter of miR-663 is hypermethylated in Chinese pediatric acute myeloid leukemia (AML). *BMC Med. Genet.* **2013**, *14*, 74. [CrossRef] [PubMed]
69. Bi, C.; Chung, T.H.; Huang, G.; Zhou, J.; Yan, J.; Ahmann, G.J.; Fonseca, R.; Chng, W.J. Genome-wide pharmacologic unmasking identifies tumor suppressive microRNAs in multiple myeloma. *Oncotarget* **2015**, *6*, 26508–26518. [CrossRef] [PubMed]
70. Jian, P.; Li, Z.W.; Fang, T.Y.; Jian, W.; Zhuan, Z.; Mei, L.X.; Yan, W.S.; Jian, N. Retinoic acid induces HL-60 cell differentiation via the upregulation of miR-663. *J. Hematol. Oncol.* **2011**, *4*, 20. [CrossRef] [PubMed]
71. Carden, T.; Singh, B.; Mooga, V.; Bajpai, P.; Singh, K.K. Epigenetic modification of miR-663 controls mitochondria-to-nucleus retrograde signaling and tumor progression. *J. Biol. Chem.* **2017**, *292*, 20694–20706. [CrossRef] [PubMed]
72. Schiedel, M.; Robaa, D.; Rumpf, T.; Sippl, W.; Jung, M. The Current State of NAD$^+$—Dependent Histone Deacetylases (Sirtuins) as Novel Therapeutic Targets. *Med. Res. Rev.* **2018**, *38*, 147–200. [CrossRef] [PubMed]
73. Kumar, S.; Kim, C.W.; Simmons, R.D.; Jo, H. Role of flow-sensitive microRNAs in endothelial dysfunction and atherosclerosis: Mechanosensitive athero-miRs. *Arterioscler. Thromb. Vasc. Biol.* **2014**, *34*, 2206–2216. [CrossRef] [PubMed]
74. Ni, C.W.; Qiu, H.; Jo, H. MicroRNA-663 upregulated by oscillatory shear stress plays a role in inflammatory response of endothelial cells. *Am. J. Physiol. Heart Circ. Physiol.* **2011**, *300*, H1762–H1769. [CrossRef] [PubMed]
75. Afonyushkin, T.; Oskolkova, O.V.; Bochkov, V.N. Permissive role of miR-663 in induction of VEGF and activation of the ATF4 branch of unfolded protein response in endothelial cells by oxidized phospholipids. *Atherosclerosis* **2012**, *225*, 50–55. [CrossRef] [PubMed]
76. Hong, Q.; Yu, S.; Geng, X.; Duan, L.; Zheng, W.; Fan, M.; Chen, X.; Wu, D. High Concentrations of Uric Acid Inhibit Endothelial Cell Migration via miR-663 Which Regulates Phosphatase and Tensin Homolog by Targeting Transforming Growth Factor-β1. *Microcirculation* **2015**, *22*, 306–314. [CrossRef] [PubMed]
77. Li, P.; Zhu, N.; Yi, B.; Wang, N.; Chen, M.; You, X.; Zhao, X.; Solomides, C.C.; Qin, Y.; Sun, J. MicroRNA-663 regulates human vascular smooth muscle cell phenotypic switch and vascular neointimal formation. *Circ. Res.* **2013**, *113*, 1117–1127. [CrossRef] [PubMed]
78. Kalani, M.; Hodjati, H.; GhamarTalepoor, A.; Samsami Dehaghani, A.; Doroudchi, M. CagA-positive and CagA-negative Helicobacter pylori strains differentially affect the expression of micro RNAs 21, 92a, 155 and 663 in human umbilical vein endothelial cells. *Cell. Mol. Biol.* **2017**, *63*, 34–40. [CrossRef] [PubMed]
79. Yang, L.; Pang, Y.; Moses, H.L. TGF-β and immune cells: An important regulatory axis in the tumor microenvironment and progression. *Trends Immunol.* **2010**, *31*, 220–227. [CrossRef] [PubMed]

80. Li, D.P.; Fan, J.; Wu, Y.J.; Xie, Y.F.; Zha, J.M.; Zhou, X.M. MiR-155 up-regulated by TGF-β promotes epithelial-mesenchymal transition, invasion and metastasis of human hepatocellular carcinoma cells in vitro. *Am. J. Trans. Res.* **2017**, *9*, 2956–2965.
81. Lin, X.; Zhen, X.; Huang, H.; Wu, H.; You, Y.; Guo, P.; Gu, X.; Yang, F. Role of MiR-155 Signal Pathway in Regulating Podocyte Injury Induced by TGF-β1. *Cell. Physiol. Biochem.* **2017**, *42*, 1469–1480. [CrossRef] [PubMed]

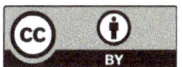

© 2018 by the authors. Licensee MDPI, Basel, Switzerland. This article is an open access article distributed under the terms and conditions of the Creative Commons Attribution (CC BY) license (http://creativecommons.org/licenses/by/4.0/).

MDPI
St. Alban-Anlage 66
4052 Basel
Switzerland
Tel. +41 61 683 77 34
Fax +41 61 302 89 18
www.mdpi.com

Medicines Editorial Office
E-mail: medicines@mdpi.com
www.mdpi.com/journal/medicines

www.ingramcontent.com/pod-product-compliance
Lightning Source LLC
LaVergne TN
LVHW071958080526
838202LV00064B/6781